T0325162

Rethinking Evidence in the Time of Pandemics

Rethinking Evidence in the Time of Pandemics

Scientific vs Narrative Rationality
and Medical Knowledge Practices

Eivind Engebretsen
University of Oslo

Mona Baker
University of Oslo

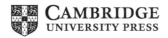

CAMBRIDGE
UNIVERSITY PRESS

University Printing House, Cambridge CB2 8BS, United Kingdom

One Liberty Plaza, 20th Floor, New York, NY 10006, USA

477 Williamstown Road, Port Melbourne, VIC 3207, Australia

314–321, 3rd Floor, Plot 3, Splendor Forum, Jasola District Centre,
New Delhi – 110025, India

103 Penang Road, #05–06/07, Visioncrest Commercial, Singapore 238467

Cambridge University Press is part of the University of Cambridge.

It furthers the University's mission by disseminating knowledge in the pursuit of
education, learning, and research at the highest international levels of excellence.

www.cambridge.org
Information on this title: www.cambridge.org/9781316516607
DOI: 10.1017/9781009030687

First published 2022

A catalogue record for this publication is available from the British Library.

ISBN 978-1-316-51660-7 Hardback

....

Contents

Tables and Figures

Acknowledgements

This book was initiated in the context of *The Body in Translation: Historicising and Reinventing Medical Humanities and Knowledge Translation*, an international research project led by Eivind Engebretsen and John Ødemark and based at the Centre for Advanced Study, the Norwegian Academy of Science and Letters in Oslo during the academic year 2019/2020. We are grateful to the Centre for its hospitality and support, which were invaluable during the early phase of developing the plan of the book, and for providing the funding for open-access publication of the final manuscript. A special thanks to Professor John Ødemark, co-PI of the *The Body in Translation*, for his continued support.

We would also like to acknowledge the support of the Centre for Sustainable Healthcare Education (SHE) at the Faculty of Medicine, University of Oslo, with which we are both affiliated. We thank SHE for co-funding the project and members of the research group Knowledge in Translation (KNOWIT) for their input to and feedback on the general arguments outlined in this publication.

Finally, we would like to express our gratitude to our editors at Cambridge University Press, Anna Whiting and Camille Lee-Own, for their professionalism and unfailing support during the writing of this manuscript.

Evidence in Times of Crisis

In a highly critical review of Carl Zimmer's *A Planet of Viruses*, Carr (2021) poses an important question: 'Is science a single, universal process that stands apart from struggles for power and resources – aka politics? Or is science the name for multiple processes, undertaken by different groups of people for different goals, all conducted in the very trenches of political struggle?' Among Carr's misgivings about *A Planet of Viruses* is that it tells half a story – the half that is devoid of politics. For instance, 'we learn how pathologists figured out that HIV comes from a primate virus', but not why so many gay people died from AIDS. What role did actors other than the virus play in this process – for instance, the Reagan administration's decision to block federal funding for HIV research? Likewise, Zimmer's account of the almost complete wipeout of Native Americans by smallpox attributes this disaster to the natives' 'immunological naivete with respect to the Europeans' accidental viral transmission', ignoring extensive scholarly work which maintains that it was essentially 'the violently imposed infrastructures of settler colonialism' that created the conditions within which the smallpox pandemic emerged and spread.

Meanwhile, the coronavirus (Covid-19) crisis that has engulfed all societies and dominated our thinking since the end of 2019 has placed the relationship between science and politics at centre stage. The repeated claim by many political leaders that they are 'following the science' as they make decisions that affect the lives of millions of people has come under attack for various reasons. Smith (2021) argues that this claim discourages citizens from thinking for themselves, because it suggests that science speaks with one voice; that it is a monolith; and hence that there is no room or need to debate its findings. But clearly science does not speak with one voice. It also rarely offers unequivocal answers, and its findings require time to verify. Cayley (2020) further suggests that viewing science as a monolith disables it, turns it into 'a pompous oracle that speaks in a single mighty voice', and at the same time 'cripples policy':

> Rather than admitting to the judgments they have made, politicians shelter behind the skirts of science. This allows them to appear valiant – they are fearlessly following science – while at the same time absolving them of responsibility for the choices they have actually made or failed to make.

Policy responses to the identification and rapid spread of the highly mutated severe acute respiratory syndrome coronavirus 2 (SARS-CoV-2) variant Omicron in November 2021 brought the tension and entanglement between science and politics into sharp focus. While politicians responded to this new threat by imposing extensive border bans, especially on flights from African countries where the variant was first identified and where it was assumed to have originated, scientists disagreed about the efficacy and timing of such measures. Some maintained that it was too late to impose such bans as the variant had already been identified in numerous countries and was circulating globally within days of it being reported by South Africa. Others argued that targeted border controls might discourage countries from reporting future variants. Others still pointed out that restrictions on commercial flights disrupt scientific work by blocking the transport of laboratory supplies needed for sequencing, hence impacting the speed with which new variants may be investigated. On 2 December, less than two weeks after the first travel bans were announced, a bioinformatician in South Africa told *Nature*: 'By next week, if nothing changes, we will run out of sequencing reagents' (Mallapaty 2021). And finally, recalling the issue of the entanglement of science and politics raised by Carr (2021), an article published in *Al-Jazeera* on 6 December argued that the bans on South Africa and neighbouring countries 'do not reflect a sound public health policy' but rather reveal the persistence of a colonial mindset that continues to shape the relationship between Europe and Africa (Kagumire 2021). Tilley (2020:161), on whose research the *Al-Jazeera* article draws, recalls that by the early twentieth century European colonizers had subjected many African cities to 'race-based segregation strategies', informed by germ theory, that were defended on the basis that they would 'keep "white" officials healthier and separate them from infected African "carriers"'. The colonial overtones of medical and political practices continue to haunt us and challenge the idea that science and politics are two separate realms.

This book views science as inevitably and inextricably embedded in a multitude of narratives such as those told by Zimmer, Carr, Kagumire and numerous others, both scientists and non-scientists. We acknowledge, moreover, that scientific claims are themselves narratives, and that whatever their factual status, they are ultimately assessed on the basis of people's lived experience and the values they hold most dear. We try to tell multiple stories from a variety of perspectives and offer a theoretical basis for understanding how different individuals and communities decide which of a range of competing stories they should believe in and why. The theoretical framework we apply assumes that understanding intricate scientific details is not an innate skill, but telling and assessing narratives is. If it wasn't, none of us would be able to engage with the multitude of stories that make up our social world or make decisions about how to act, and on what basis. While accepting that scientific evidence has a key role to play in shaping public policy and should – in an ideal world – be taken seriously by members of the public, we demonstrate through numerous examples that it is often mistrusted and/or overridden by considerations that are affective and social in nature. These considerations, in turn, are informed by the narratives to which we are all socialized over many years and in numerous contexts.

The Covid-19 crisis offers many resonant examples that allow us to flesh out and demonstrate the theoretical principles that inform our arguments. But the scope of our argument is much broader than Covid-19, and broader even than pandemics as such. In developing an approach to medical knowledge that can account for the way both experts and non-experts make sense of what constitutes reliable evidence in various contexts, we are not merely concerned with the *science* of Covid-19 or pandemics but with the myriad discourses in which different narrators articulate their understanding and evaluation of different types of evidence, whether or not they draw on scientific sources. Our point of departure is Walter Fisher's distinction (outlined in Chapter 2) between the world as 'a set of logical puzzles that can be solved through appropriate analysis and application of reason conceived as an argumentative construct' (Fisher 1987:59), and the world as 'a set of stories that must be chosen among to live the good life in a process of continual recreation' (Fisher 1984:8). We engage with this distinction specifically as it plays out in the field of medicine, and in the recent Covid-19 crisis, but we believe that it provides a helpful point of departure in examining many other areas of social and cultural life. Rather than treating various practices of knowledge as rational or irrational in purely scientific terms, we attempt to understand the controversies surrounding Covid-19, as a case in point, by drawing on a theoretical framework that recognizes and explains different types of rationality, and hence plural conceptualizations of evidence.

Some of the issues we raise are exemplified by the controversy reported in *The New York Times* in August 2020 under the title 'The Covid drug wars that pitted doctor vs doctor' (Dominus 2020). The question which 'opened up a civil war' between clinicians drawing on their experience to save lives and medical researchers who believe that '[r]elying on gut instinct rather than evidence . . . was essentially "witchcraft"' is: 'How much freedom should front-line clinicians have in treating Covid-19 with unproven drugs'. The *New York Times* report, which involved interviewing several clinicians, reveals that the issue is much more complex than the question suggests. Even physicians who had been committed to relying on evidence from randomized controlled trials (RCTs), according to colleagues, wanted access to all types of unproven medicines when it was their mother fighting for her life. For decisions that directly affect us or our loved ones, scientific evidence may be largely overridden by other considerations, even for those who would otherwise appeal to it as the only rational basis for decision making.

1.1 The Status of Evidence in Evidence-Based Medicine

The Covid-19 crisis has transformed the highly specialized issue of what constitutes reliable medical evidence into a topic of public concern. Newspapers and social media abound with discussions about whether the evidence for wearing masks is weak or strong, or whether mass public health measures such as lockdowns or school closures are backed by sufficient evidence. At the same time, a global initiative for gathering evidence to support the development of new, more effective vaccines and drugs continues in laboratories and clinics that are far removed from these sites of public debate and from the immediate pressure of delivering healthcare in emergency situations. Underpinning all these different discussions about and approaches to evidence is a shared assumption: that evidence is singular and that it can be ranked on a singular scale as present or absent, strong or weak, from a purely rational, value-free perspective. This book interrogates the assumption that evidence means the same thing to different constituencies and in different contexts by outlining a more nuanced and socially responsive approach to medical expertise that incorporates scientific and lay processes of making sense of the world and deciding how to act in it. In so doing, it hopes to provide a point of orientation for clinicians working at the coalface, whose experience is sometimes at odds with the type of rationality that underpins evidence-based medicine (EBM) and that guides researchers conducting RCTs. The argument elaborated also has implications for policy makers in the healthcare system, who have to navigate similar pressures and contradictions between scientific and lay rationality to produce meaningful guidelines in the midst of a runaway pandemic.

While using Covid-19 as an exemplary case study, this book takes as its point of departure the premise that the controversies surrounding the nature of evidence were also present in earlier epidemics such as SARS and Ebola virus, and that they will continue to plague our responses to future pandemics unless we learn to address them more effectively.

Pandemics in general, and Covid-19 in particular, are emblematic sites for exploring and challenging concepts of evidence because they clearly transform such concepts into a topic of public concern and demonstrate the relevance and urgency of engaging with the processes by which they come to be understood and assessed differently by various constituencies.

In medicine and healthcare, the EBM paradigm, which started to emerge in the 1990s, has contributed to promoting an understanding of evidence as a singular phenomenon that can be ranked on a singular scale. According to Sackett et al.'s (1996) much cited definition, EBM is 'the conscientious, explicit and judicious use of current best evidence in making decisions about the care of individual patients'. In line with this programmatic statement, EBM has emphasized the use of clinical guidelines and challenged clinicians to question their reliance on pathophysiological reasoning and unenhanced clinical judgement. Clinicians are now trained in reading research literature and converting the findings from published studies into probabilities based on mathematical estimates (Solomon 2015). Accordingly, the EBM movement has developed mathematical and experimental techniques for producing and evaluating evidence, including statistical meta-analysis of research results and methods for developing and implementing clinical guideline recommendations.

The framework EBM developed for ranking evidence rests on a hierarchy that features simple observational methods at the bottom and moves on to increasingly rigorous methodologies, notably comparative experimental intervention studies, RCTs and systematic reviews of such trials at the top of the evidence pyramid. Although this hierarchy has been criticized and modified, a dominant assumption among EBM advocates is still that findings generated by RCTs are likely to be 'closer to the true effect than the findings generated by other research methods' (Evans 2003:78). Epistemologically, the EBM hierarchy relies on observations (empiricism) as the method of knowing; ontologically, it conceives of reality as a set of causal mechanisms (realism) (Greenhalgh et al. 2014; Engebretsen et al. 2016). But as the Covid-19 crisis clearly illustrates, there are many sites of knowledge construction in medicine – let alone other spheres of practice – where these rules do not apply. Recovery stories, for instance, are intended to give voice to the patients' perspectives and draw on an experienced reality rather than empirical findings, while a policy brief aims to provide strategies and points to a reality of ideas and visions rather than of embodied practices. While also engaging with the type of knowledge elaborated in discourses such as policy briefs and patient statements, the EBM evidence hierarchy only acknowledges one single concept of evidence, that is, 'close to the true effect'. Hence, the EBM conception of knowledge fails to acknowledge that the way different groups engage in the process of knowing – as articulated in different types of discourse – determines the principles and objects of their knowledge.

The narrative framework that informs our analysis of how medical researchers, medical practitioners, policy makers and lay people conceptualize and evaluate evidence recognizes that 'human beings are as much valuing as they are reasoning beings' (Fisher 1997:314). In outlining and extending this framework, we seek not only to interrogate current, restricted conceptualizations of evidence in the EBM model, but also to elaborate a more socially responsive approach to expertise that can offer insight into the sources of controversy around medical phenomena such as Covid-19 and a more productive approach to addressing them and communicating medical information without unduly antagonizing large swathes of the population. The scheme we offer is largely diagnostic, although we argue in Chapter 6 that we also have a moral responsibility to introduce creative possibilities in our interaction with others by constructing narratives that "provoke intellectual struggle . . . and the creation of a more workable human order" (Bennett and Edelman 1985:162; Baker 2006:163). As far as medical controversies are concerned, we do not offer recommendations but rather a model of analysis that can shed light on why different people arrive at different decisions based on the same sources of evidence, and why we must acknowledge their reasons for doing so as rooted in different types of rationality rather than dismissing them as irrational. Ultimately, as Fisher (1987:113) explains, the purpose of the narrative paradigm we apply throughout this book is 'to ensure that people are conscious of the values they adhere to and would promote in rhetorical transactions, and to inform their consciousness *without dictating what they should believe*' (emphasis in original).

This book shares some of the theoretical assumptions of narrative medicine, but it also differs from the large body of scholarship in that field in important ways. While narrative medicine is mainly concerned with clinical practice, the model we introduce extends to the daily lives of all citizens and the way in which knowledge based on medical evidence is accepted or rejected by all members of society. On a conceptual level, our approach does not rely on the distinction – inherent in narrative medicine – between narrative medicine as the 'art' and EBM as the 'science' of medical practice (Solomon 2015:178). From the perspective of the narrative paradigm, EBM is embedded in a multiplicity of narratives and hence is itself 'an interpretation of some aspect of the world that is historically and culturally grounded and shaped by human personality' (Fisher 1987:49). Importantly, we do not reject the EBM paradigm, nor do we suggest that it should be replaced by the narrative paradigm. We merely argue that – from the perspective of the narrative paradigm – the empiricist notion of evidence underpinning EBM is only one possible situated interpretation or value according to which knowledge claims can be and are in practice assessed. This means that the narrative paradigm is not a practical tool for improving medicine but rather an epistemological tool that reveals the values on the basis of which we assess stories and claims of evidence. By contrast with the narrative paradigm framework proposed here, narrative medicine does focus on improving medicine and is fundamentally linked to the idea of caring for the individual patient. Solomon (2015) distinguishes four general aspects of narrative medicine as it has evolved since the late 1980s: (1) listening and attentiveness to the patient's story and point of view; (2) empathy or experiential understanding of what the patient is going through; (3) detective work or attention to the explicit and implicit contents of the patient's story; and (4) meaning making or the act of making sense of the patient's sufferings through storytelling, for example through narratives of restitution, chaos and redemption (Frank 1995). Our aim is different: we draw on and adapt the narrative paradigm in order to provide a framework for understanding how we assess different narratives on the basis of the values we believe each encodes and the extent to which they resonate with our own values and beliefs.

1.2 Organization of Chapters

Chapter 2, 'Narrative Rationality and the Logic of Good Reasons', outlines the main tenets of the narrative paradigm, acknowledges critical scholarship relating to its applicability in some cases and settings, and demonstrates its usefulness through a variety of examples from different areas of controversy that arose during the Covid-19 pandemic and are dealt with in more detail in chapters 3, 4 and 5. The chapters that follow do not only explain different antagonisms surrounding Covid-19 from the perspective of the narrative paradigm as elaborated by Walter Fisher, but also extend the framework. They nuance the narrative paradigm in the course of analysis, especially with reference to its application to medical narratives and its potential for offering a point of orientation for medical practitioners and policy makers in the healthcare sector.

Arguments about the pros and cons and possible effectiveness of face masks have occupied considerable space in specialist, medical venues such as peer-reviewed journals and science blogs as well as public forums such as mainstream media and social media – the latter attracting contributions from medical specialists and lay members of the public alike. The debate has often been heated, and there have also been reports of individuals resisting the stipulation to wear face masks in shops and on airplanes, at times leading to acts of physical violence. Drawing on the theoretical model outlined in Chapter 2, Chapter 3, 'Whose Evidence? What Rationality? The Face Mask Controversy', examines some of the arguments for and against face masks as articulated by a diverse range of individuals and constituencies, within and beyond the Anglophone and European world, and the justifications given in each case, as well as the underlying values and logics of these various parties.

Chapter 4, 'Whose Lives? What Values? Herd Immunity, Lockdowns, and Social/ Physical Distancing', examines disagreements about mass public health measures such as lockdowns and physical distancing, which have dominated discussions around Covid-19. Policy-oriented discourses such as recommendations and media briefings have argued for more or less severe measures, ranging from national curfews to mandated physical distancing (unfortunately termed social distancing) or mitigation strategies built on the premise of quickly reaching herd immunity. All these different measures have been extensively debated in the media and other public forums and continuously monitored by international organizations such as the World Health Organization. Policy arguments have also been revised or refocused in tandem with a growing body of research and natural experiments as countries began to introduce either mandatory or voluntary policies. Chapter 4 examines various arguments deployed in this debate and the complex dialogue between political, scientific and popular values and discourses.

Chapter 5, 'The Rational World Paradigm, the Narrative Paradigm and the Politics of Pharmaceutical Intervention', examines some of the rationales for pharmaceutical interventions, especially vaccines, and resistance to them. Vaccine-hesitant and anti-vaccine activists have questioned different aspects of the Covid-19 vaccination programme, and some have even argued that the whole virus is a scam and part of a plot to profit from selling vaccines. The discussion regarding vaccines and other potential pharmaceutical treatments quickly became highly politicized, especially after Donald Trump's official endorsement of the malaria drug hydroxychloroquine. The debate about vaccines and treatments does not only reflect tensions between science and politics and expert and non-expert discourses. It also highlights the fact that there are divergent views within the scientific community itself on when new evidence may be ready to be put into political action. Chapter 5 explores the divergent arguments used in this debate as well as their various and complex value-laden underpinnings.

In the final chapter, 'Objectivist vs Praxial Knowledge: Towards a Model of Situated Epistemologies and Narrative Identification, we revisit some of the tenets of the narrative paradigm, based on the analyses presented in the preceding three chapters, and suggest ways in which the concept of narrative rationality may be further developed and nuanced. Fisher distinguishes between objectivist knowledge and praxial knowledge, and argues that it is the latter type of knowledge that narrative rationality seeks to 'foster and support' (Fisher 1994:26). The aim of Chapter 6 is to use this distinction as a starting point to develop a model for situated epistemologies based on insights drawn from Fisher's narrative paradigm, proposals put forward by some of his critics and the work of thinkers such as Heidegger and Kristeva, together with more recent work on narrativity.

Narrative Rationality and the Logic of Good Reasons

This chapter provides a theoretical basis for examining the tension between scientific and lay rationality that continues to undermine attempts to address such vital healthcare issues as vaccine hesitancy (Larson 2020) or lack of compliance with regulations and test regimes during a pandemic (Fancourt et al. 2020). Rather than treating different responses and attitudes towards particular issues as rational or irrational in purely scientific terms, the theoretical framework we discuss here acknowledges different types of rationality, and hence plural conceptualizations of evidence. In outlining this framework, the aim is to elaborate a nuanced and socially responsive approach to expertise and knowledge – an approach that can offer insight into the sources of controversy around medical phenomena such as Covid-19 and a more productive means of communicating medical information.

2.1 The Narrative Paradigm: Basic Tenets

The basic assumption underpinning what has come to be known as the narrative paradigm is that '[n]o matter how strictly a case is argued – scientifically, philosophically, or legally – it will always be a story, an interpretation of some aspect of the world that is historically and culturally grounded and shaped by human personality' (Fisher 1987:49). Even a scientific argument or claim, however abstract, is ultimately processed as a story and interpreted not in isolation but as part of a particular narrative take on the world. In this sense, all knowledge is 'ultimately configured narratively, as a component in a larger story implying the being of a certain kind of person, a person with a particular world view, with a specific self-concept, and with characteristic ways of relating to others' (Fisher 1987:17).

Importantly, our embeddedness in the narratives that constitute our world and within which we live our lives does not preclude an ability to reflect on, question and assess these narratives. We assess the narratives that surround us against the principles of *coherence* and *fidelity*, as discussed in detail later in this chapter. As such, we are all 'full participants in the making of a message', whether we are authors or audience members (Fisher 1987:18). The narrative paradigm suggests that we ultimately assess different versions of competing narratives on the basis of the values we believe each encodes and the extent to which they resonate with our own values and beliefs. This explains, for instance, the diametrically opposed responses we have witnessed to scientific arguments about the need to wear a face mask during the Covid crisis (see Chapter 3). On the one hand, these arguments are vocally rejected by some on the basis that the mandate to wear a mask encroaches on their personal freedom and is a form of control over their bodies; at the same time, others accept the mandate willingly and see compliance with it as a matter of moral responsibility to protect themselves and those they may come into contact with. Neither group can simply be dismissed as irrational. The narrative paradigm attempts to make sense of such responses through the concept of narrative rationality, understood as a '"logic" intrinsic to the very idea of narrativity' (Fisher 1985b:87). Narrative rationality asserts that 'it is not the *individual form* of argument that is ultimately persuasive in discourse. That is important, but *values* are more persuasive, and they may be expressed in a variety of modes, of which argument is only one' (Fisher 1987:48; emphasis in original). Greenhalgh (2016:3) makes a similar point in the context of using narrative research in healthcare when she argues that '[s]tories convince not by their objective truth but by their likeness to real life and their emotional impact on the reader or listener'.

This is not the same as arguing that all knowledge is equally rational or true, or that any 'good reason' (in Fisher's terms, as discussed below) is as good as another. The concept of narrative rationality merely suggests that 'whatever is taken as a basis for adopting a rhetorical message is inextricably bound to a value – to a conception of the good' (Fisher 1987:107). Whether originating in a transcendental belief in universal human rights or in adherence to a specific religious stipulation, 'a value is valuable not because it is tied to a reason or is expressed by a reasonable person per se, but because *it makes a pragmatic difference in one's life and in one's community*' (Fisher 1987:111; emphasis in original). It follows, then, that it is only by creating awareness about the specific values people adhere to and invest in their narratives that we can adequately understand why they believe in these particular stories. As such, the narrative paradigm provides a radical democratic ground for social political critique (Fisher 1987). It refutes the assumption that rationality is a privilege of the few and the exclusive possession of 'experts' who (a) have specialized knowledge about the issue at hand, (b) are cognizant of the argumentative procedures dominant within the field, and (c) weigh all arguments in a systematic and deliberative fashion (Fisher 1987). From the perspective of the narrative paradigm, all human beings are rational. While technical concepts and criteria for judging the rationality of communication can be highly valuable in the specialized contexts in which these concepts are developed, they do not represent absolute standards of truth. No community, knowledge or genres can have a final claim to such standards. Moreover, as soon as the expert 'crosses the boundary of technical knowledge into the territory of life as it ought to be lived' (Fisher 1987:73), he or she becomes subject to the demands of narrative rationality. When the medical expert, for instance, engages in public discourse regarding pandemic-related measures or in dialogue with patients about everyday health problems, he or she is obliged to leave the rationality of their technical community and submit to the narrative criteria for 'determining whose story is most coherent and reliable as a guide to belief and action' (Fisher 1984:13). Such a democratic understanding is a prerequisite to elaborating effective narratives that can enhance the reception of medical knowledge and reduce some of the sources of resistance and misunderstanding that continue to plague public communication during critical events such as pandemics.

The starting point for the narrative paradigm is that storytelling is *the* defining feature of humanity; we are *homo narrans* (narrating humans) before being *homo sapiens* (wise or knowing humans). The *homo narrans* metaphor is central to the narrative paradigm: it shifts the focus to the everyday, pre-reflective, practical aspect of being in the world in Heideggerian terms. The assumption is that it is 'through our practical engagement with the world that a thing becomes what it is' (Qvortrup and Nielsen 2019:149). Because we dwell in narratives, we respond to (communicative) experiences instinctively before we begin to evaluate them consciously. Indeed, the narrative paradigm assumes that rationality itself 'is born out of something prerational, an experience that in the very moment defies classification and explanation, but delivers us something to classify or explain after the fact' (Qvortrup and Nielsen 2019:156). While traditional rationality is a skill that has to be actively learned and cultivated and – importantly – involves a high degree of self-consciousness, 'the narrative impulse is part of our very being because we acquire narrativity in the natural process of socialization' (Fisher 1987:65). The narrative paradigm thus offers a way of conceptualizing the world in which 'practice precedes theory' (Qvortrup and Nielsen 2019:149), and indeed Fisher presents narrative rationality as 'an attempt to recapture Aristotle's concept of *phronesis*', or practical wisdom (Fisher 1985a:350; emphasis in original). In the context of healthcare, the narrative paradigm suggests that clinicians are instinctively guided first by the narratives they have come to subscribe to over time, some of which arise from their practical experience of delivering healthcare, and only secondarily by the evidence from controlled trials and other theoretically informed data. The same is true of a significant proportion of frontline healthcare workers in England (mostly black and ethnic minorities) who continued to turn down the offer of vaccination when it was introduced in early 2021 (Sample 2021), despite having the same access to arguments explaining the importance of vaccination as their white colleagues (see Chapter 5 for a fuller discussion of this issue). Lay members of the public similarly adopt or shun the healthcare options available to them on the basis of how they fit into the narratives to which they subscribe and that constitute their sense of self, rather than on the basis of scientific evidence that they cannot, at any rate, directly assess for themselves. Ultimately, the logic of narrative rationality 'entails a reconceptualization of knowledge, one that permits the possibility of wisdom' (Fisher 1994:21).[1]

In understanding the scope of this claim, and some critiques of it discussed in the literature (e.g., Kirkwood 1992; see Chapter 6 for details), it is important to note the difference Fisher draws between narrative as paradigm and narrative as mode of discourse. 'The narrative paradigm', he explains, 'is a paradigm in the sense that it expresses and implies a philosophical view of human communication; it is not a model of discourse as such' (Fisher 1987:90). Narration here is to be understood as a conceptual framework rather than a text type or genre. It is also not a retroactive discursive phenomenon, that is, the act of telling a story, but a metaphor for living (Qvortrup and Nielsen 2019:152). Rather than seeing narratives as temporal wholes consisting of a beginning, a middle and an end, the narrative paradigm considers narration as an open-ended possibility. While the philosophical ground of the rational world paradigm is epistemology, that of the narrative paradigm is ontology (Qvortrup and Nielsen 2019:146). The rational world paradigm functions through 'self-evident propositions, demonstrations, and proofs, the verbal expressions of certain and probable knowing' (Fisher 1984:4). The narrative paradigm, on the other hand, is concerned with the primary mode of being in the

---

[1] The narrative paradigm draws on the original conception of logos in ancient Greece, a conception Fisher traces back to Isocrates and his work *Antidosis*, which encompasses both story and reason and 'outward and inward thought' (Fisher 1987:13). Logos, as understood in the ancient world, was not the territory of a privileged discourse: 'all communicative behaviour was presumed to be rational, although not necessarily in the same way' (Fisher 1987:24). Fisher expands the notion of logos to include rhetoric and poetic discourse (along with philosophy and science), but he also draws on this broad conception of logos to rethink the understanding and practice of logic. Logic, he suggests, must be understood to include 'a systematic set of concepts, procedures, and criteria for determining the degree of truthfulness or certainty in human discourse' (Fisher 1987:27).

world, with the way in which we instinctively and pre-reflectively embed any experience within a story or the set of stories that constitute our world in order to make sense of it. This is different from the specific form that a given discourse might take, whether it is a novel or a scholarly paper for instance. In the paradigm (rather than mode of discourse) sense, all forms of communication ultimately contribute to and can only be understood with reference to larger societal narratives. As a mode of discourse, on the other hand, we can distinguish between narration, exposition, argumentation, and various other genres and explore their appropriateness or otherwise for communicating health and other types of knowledge. Fisher suggests, for example, that 'narration works by suggestion and identification' whereas 'argument operates by inferential moves and deliberation'; from the narrative paradigm perspective, 'the differences between them are structural rather than substantive' (Fisher 1984:15). As Roberts (2004:130–131) puts it, '[p]eople are not essentially arguers, but rather storytellers, and sometimes those narratives merely take the form of argument'.

2.2 Narrative Paradigm vs Rational World Paradigm

Before we discuss how the narrative paradigm might help us appreciate some of the tensions and concerns that continue to hamper the delivery of healthcare in many contexts, it is useful to explain how it differs from the type of rationality traditionally used to assess arguments and responses to them, including in medical and scientific contexts.

The narrative paradigm assumes that all human beings are capable of reasoning, irrespective of their level of education or training. In some ways, society already acknowledges the inherent (narrative) rationality of all humans, their innate practical wisdom: it does so when it appoints lay members of the public to juries that have the power to decide the fate of defendants, and when it acknowledges the right of all citizens to vote in elections, irrespective of their background or education. In such contexts, truth is associated with identification, not deliberation – with what 'rings true' among voters and members of the public. In most other contexts, however, rationality is associated with a scientific, empirical approach to knowledge, which assumes that (educated) people are able to assess arguments by applying the standards of formal and informal logic. This view of rationality focuses on the world as a set of puzzles that can be solved through inferential analysis and 'empirical investigations tied to such systems as "cost-benefit" analysis'. 'Method, techniques and technology' are the means used by this type of rationality to solve problems; 'efficiency, productivity, power, and effectiveness are its values' (Fisher 1994:25). True knowledge is understood to be objective: 'the result of observation, description, explanation, prediction, and control' (Fisher 1994:25). In medicine, this type of rationality is often frequency-based, in the belief that '"although we can't predict the future for the individual case, we can be 'usually' right (eg, 95% of the time)" as long as events or cases are frequent enough' (Wieringa et al. 2018a:88; citing Hacking 2001). Healthcare decisions, the argument goes, should therefore be guided by large amounts of data, ideally collected through systematic reviews of randomized controlled trials (RCTs). Fisher asserts that this scientific, empirical view of rationality 'informs the mind-set of researchers and consultants for virtually all levels of decision making in every social, political, educational, legislative, and business institution in society' (Fisher 1994:25). It constitutes the dominant way of understanding reason that has prevailed in the Western tradition since Plato: as 'an achievement of training, skill, or education' (Stroud 2016:1). In medicine, it has reached its point of culmination in the evidence-based medicine (EBM) paradigm, which argues that healthcare decisions should be grounded in high-quality medical research. EBM provides tools to distinguish between high- and low-quality evidence and to appraise research evidence based on scientific rationality (see Chapters 1 and 6 for a more detailed discussion). The knowledge produced by this type of rationality tells us what is 'instrumentally feasible and profitable' but not how to address issues of justice, happiness and humanity (Fisher 1994:25). It is 'knowledge of that' and 'knowledge of how' but not 'knowledge of whether' (Fisher 1994:25); it 'gives one power but not discretion' and 'drive[s] out wisdom' (Fisher 1994:26):

> Medical doctors *know that* by using certain technological devices they can keep one alive even when the brain is 'dead', They *know how* to do this. The question of *whether* they do this is beyond their science. . . . Doctors and scientists, as *technicians*, may dismiss, ignore, or relegate this sort of knowledge to others – it is not their business – but they cannot do so without denying their humanity.[2] (Fisher 1994:25; emphasis in original)

At the point where medical doctors cross the boundary of technical knowledge – where knowing that and knowing how dominate – and enter 'the territory of life as it ought to be lived' (Fisher 1987:73), they are 'off-duty'. They then pass from the domain of facts to the domain of values, from what they *know* to what they should *do* (Lonergan 1992; Engebretsen et al. 2015). Questions such as *whether* to impose lockdowns or make vaccination mandatory are not strictly scientific but political. In relation to such questions, the expert takes on the role of a counsellor 'which is, as Walter Benjamin notes, the true function of the storyteller' (Fisher 1987:73). Outside the controlled context of an experiment or trial, practical problems also become the focal point for competing expert stories that address the issue from different angles. The question of whether or not to impose lockdowns or make vaccination mandatory, for instance, might be framed very differently from the point of view of immunologists, psychiatrists, sociologists and educational scientists. The narrative paradigm asserts that none of these experts can 'pronounce a story that ends all storytelling' (Fisher 1987:73).[3]

Narrative rationality attempts to combine knowledge of *that* and knowledge of *how* with knowledge of *whether*, and supplements them with 'a praxial consciousness' (Fisher 1994:25). Because values are central to this view of rationality, the operative principle of the narrative paradigm is '*identification* rather than deliberation' (Fisher 1987:66; emphasis in original). Thus, for example, despite being 'told from a subordinate position in the knowledge hierarchy', narratives of natural childbirth that draw on 'subjective, experiential and visceral knowledge' (Susam-Sarajeva 2020:47, 48) can challenge institutional narratives of progress, science and modernity precisely because they persuade through identification rather than logical argumentation. In the words of Ina May Gaskin, author of *Ina May's Guide to Childbirth*,

> [stories] teach us the occasional difference between accepted medical knowledge and the real bodily experiences that women have – including those that are never reported in medical textbooks nor admitted as possibilities in the medical world. . . . Birth stories told by women who were active participants in giving birth often express a good deal of practical wisdom, inspiration, and information for other women.
> (Gaskin 2003, cited in Susam Sarajeva 2020:48)

---

[2] Fisher acknowledges that 'many doctors and scientists are keenly aware of this fact' (Fisher 1994:25).
[3] Stengers (2013) also discusses the difference between practical problems and scientific problems, the role of experts and the question of who owns the problem in some detail.

Hollihan and Riley's study of parents of difficult children, who came together in a network of parental support called 'Toughlove', found that participants felt that the 'rational world, with its scientific notions of child-psychology . . . did not speak to them' (Hollihan and Riley 1987:23), whereas the Toughlove story, which lay the blame on their children and encouraged them to adopt tough measures to discipline them, 'resonated with their own feelings that they were essentially good people whose only failing had been that they were too permissive and not as tough as their own parents had been' (Hollihan and Riley 1987: 23).

Narratives, then, compete to the extent that they are able to connect and resonate with the audience's values and sense of self; rational arguments, on the other hand, compete on the basis of the extent to which they follow the rules of logical inference. The rational world paradigm assumes that 'the primary mode of decision-making and judgments in human communication is argument' (Stroud 2016:1); the narrative paradigm posits that it is 'the provision of good reasons' (Stroud 2016:2), which, as we explain shortly, concerns the implicit and explicit values encoded in any message, whatever form that message takes. Narrative rationality assumes that all human beings are rational in the sense of being able to think and to hold views about various aspects of life; that they are 'reflective and from such reflection they make the stories of their lives and have the basis for judging narratives for and about them' (Fisher 1984:15). It explains how people come to 'feel at home (dwell) in multiple stories, imbuing subsequent actions with intrinsic meaning' (Qvortrup and Nielsen 2019:159). Narrative rationality is not dependent on argumentative competence in specialist fields nor on formal education, although Fisher does recognize that education can make us 'more sophisticated' in understanding and applying the principles of assessing narratives from the perspective of the narrative paradigm (Fisher 1984:15). In essence, however, narrative rationality has its own logic – the logic of good reasons – which ultimately subsumes rather than displaces traditional rationality (Fisher 1987:66). Table 2.1 sums up the differences between the rational world paradigm and the narrative paradigm as outlined in Fisher (1984:26, 30) and elsewhere.

Table 2.1 Rational world paradigm vs narrative paradigm

Rational world paradigm	Narrative paradigm
Humans are essentially rational beings.	Humans are essentially storytellers.
The appropriate mode of human decision making and communication is argument – discourse that features clear-cut inferential or implicative structures.	The paradigmatic mode of human decision making is 'good reasons', which vary in form among situations, genres and media of communication.
The conduct of argument is ruled by the dictates of situations – legal, scientific, legislative, public and so on.	The production and practice of good reasons are ruled by matters of history, biology, culture and character.
Rationality is determined by subject-matter knowledge, argumentative ability and skill in employing the rules of advocacy in given fields.	Rationality is determined by the nature of persons as narrative beings – their awareness of *narrative coherence*, whether a story 'hangs together', and their constant habit of testing *narrative fidelity*, whether or not the stories they experience ring true with the stories they know to be true in their lives.

Table 2.1 (cont.)

Rational world paradigm	Narrative paradigm
The world is a set of logical puzzles that can be solved through appropriate analysis and application of reason conceived as an argumentative construct.	The world as we know it is a set of stories that must be chosen among in order for us to live life in a process of continual re-creation.

2.3 Narrative Probability, Narrative Fidelity and the Logic of Good Reasons

The main purpose of Fisher's narrative paradigm is to provide a theoretical framework that can account for the way in which any communicative encounter – whether it involves a scientific theory, a fictional story or a factual account – is assessed by different individuals with different life experiences and values, not by resort to logical inference but on the basis of good reasons. Fisher (1987:48) defines good reasons as *'elements that provide warrants for accepting or adhering to the advice fostered by any form of communication that can be considered rhetorical'* (emphasis in original). By 'warrant', he means 'that which authorizes, sanctions, or justifies belief, attitude, or action' (Fisher 1987:107). The suggestion here is not that anything that 'warrants' a belief or action is good in and of itself, but only that whatever is taken as a basis for accepting a claim is 'inextricably bound to a value – to a conception of the good'. In this sense, 'values may be reasons and . . . reasons affirm values in and of themselves' (Fisher 1987).

Unlike traditional conceptualizations of reasoning, the logic of good reasons maintains that reasoning is not restricted to discourse that takes the form of argument, nor does it have to be expressed in the form of inferential structures; reasoning exists in all forms of human communication, including non-discursive ones (Fisher 1984:1). The components of the familiar logic of reasons associated with the rational world paradigm generally revolve around establishing the factual status of the elements that constitute any message, including whether certain facts have been omitted, and the patterns of reasoning adopted by the communicator; they pertain to questions of definition, justification and procedure (Fisher 1987). The logic of good reasons is at odds with traditional, technical approaches to knowledge because it acknowledges a high degree of subjectivity in assessing all forms of communication, including scientific data. When we assess a story, we decide, consciously or subconsciously, whether we can identify with and adhere to the values that underpin it. This implies subjective involvement. Fisher argues that 'the intrusion of subjectivity is not a fault' in the logic of good reasons, and that 'by making the considerations of values a systematic and self-conscious process, the logic of good reasons fills the space left open by technical logic, with its primary concern with formal relationships and certitude' (Fisher 1987:110). A good example that supports Fisher's argument is the fierce debate generated by Richard Herrnstein and Charles Murray's 1994 book *The Bell Curve*, which offers an analysis of racial differences and levels of intelligence in American Society based on IQ scores, and suggests that intelligence and cognitive ability are largely inherited. In a review of the book, more than 20 years after its first publication, Siegel (2017) expresses grave concern over its apparent, 'unfortunate' resurgence. He states that the authors' defence over the years has been 'It's in the data', and that most critics have failed to challenge it because they simply focused on its sources or reasoning. By contrast, Siegel argues that 'those points should actually take a secondary position within a thorough rebuke' of the book and its authors. Instead, he suggests, we should question the authors' motives (and hence values) by asking *why* they saw fit to investigate racial differences in the first place. 'Even if we assume the presented data trends are sound', he insists, we have to reject the book's argument because it tacitly invites its readers to prejudge individuals on the basis of race. In doing so, whatever the status of the data on which it is based, it condones prejudice. The ultimate value for Siegel, himself a supporter of big data, who founded the international conference series 'Predictive Analytics World', is that '[j]udging by way of category is the epitome of dehumanizing', and as such must be rejected outright.

The two principles that define narrative rationality and embody the logic of good reasons in Fisher's paradigm are narrative probability (what constitutes a coherent story) and, more specifically, narrative fidelity (whether a story resonates with the audience's experience and values). These may be thought of as tests that we apply – whether instinctively or through conscious reasoning – to decide whether a narrative coheres and offers good reasons for action and belief. A message that is judged by a particular audience to be high in narrative probability and narrative fidelity enhances identification and is more likely to be adopted or adhered to by members of that audience. As will become clear from the discussion below, narrative probability largely incorporates traditional forms of reasoning, allowing Fisher to assert that narrative rationality subsumes rather than displaces traditional rationality, as mentioned earlier. We discuss both principles in more detail below. In what follows, however, it is important to reiterate that the terms 'narrative' and 'story' as we use them here subsume any mode of discourse (argument, set of instructions, report on an experiment or account of a set of events), in line with the basic assumption in the narrative paradigm that 'there is no genre, including technical communication, that is not an episode in the story of life' (Fisher 1985a:347). A narrative, moreover, is not necessarily restricted to a single text or encounter but may be constructed from a variety of sources; even a story elaborated in a single text will always be part of an ongoing societal narrative.

2.3.1 Narrative Probability (Coherence)

Narrative probability or coherence concerns the internal consistency and integrity of a narrative, assessed on the basis of three considerations that are all familiar components of traditional reasoning: first, the structural makeup of the narrative, or the way it coheres internally, within its own bounds (**structural or argumentative coherence**); second, its external consistency and completeness in terms of how it differs from or accords with other stories on the same issue that we are aware of (**material coherence**); and third, its believability in terms of the consistency and reliability of the characters involved – primarily the character(s) articulating the story but also those depicted in it as sources of information or authority (**characterological coherence**).

According to Fisher (1987:88; emphasis in original), we assess structural or argumentative coherence on the basis of whether a narrative reveals contradictions within itself:

Narrative *coherence* refers to formal features of a story conceived as a discrete sequence of thought and/or action in life or literature . . . that is, it concerns whether the story coheres or "hangs together," whether or not a story is free of contradictions.

We depart from this definition in one important respect that has implications for the way we understand narrative fidelity and the logic of good reasons. Where Fisher seems to assume that narrative probability is a static quality present *in* the narrative, and that contradiction undermines the potential for adherence to a given story (as evident from the above definition), we follow Stroud (2002:387) in considering incoherence and contradiction as "potential entry points for novel ideas and values into the auditors' belief system" (see Chapter 6). This revision is important if we are to avoid the kind of circularity that results from assuming that we are locked into a system of values and can only accept new narratives if they are free of contradictions and already confirm our existing beliefs. Without internal (and external) contradictions there would be no scope for engaging an audience or introducing them to different perspectives on an issue. We would forever be locked into understandings of the world that confirm rather than productively challenge our existing beliefs and prejudices. And yet, we know that some of the most effective narratives – such as those elaborated in the Bible and the Qur'an – feature contradictory statements that believers do manage to reconcile and identify with. At the same time, despite much criticism of the narrative paradigm on the basis that it implies that successful narratives necessarily reinforce rather than challenge the values of the audience (Kirkwood 1992, Stroud 2002), there are instances in Fisher's prolific output where he seems to acknowledge a less passive role for the audience (Fisher 1985b:86):

> The narrative paradigm sees people as storytellers – authors and co-authors who creatively read and evaluate the texts of life and literature. It envisions existing institutions as providing 'plots' that are always in the process of re-creation rather than as scripts; it stresses that people are full participants in the making of messages, whether they are agents (authors) or audience members (co-authors).

If the audience is to play a part in the making of messages, rather than receiving and assessing them passively, we cannot rule out the possibility that some discrepancies and contradictions can be productive and may enhance rather than undermine narrative probability for some audiences. With this qualification in mind, we may now look at some examples of the way structural (in)coherence is assessed in practice.

Writing about the Swedish position on wearing masks in public during the Covid-19 crisis (see Chapter 3 for further details), and citing examples of towns and municipalities actually *banning* the use of face masks rather than enforcing it, Walravens and O'Shea (2021) ask "How on earth did we end up in this situation?" In their answer to this question, they cite several instances of structural incoherence in the institutional Swedish narrative of the pandemic that they suggest have led to confusion and account for the low levels of compliance on the part of the public. The story begins with the Swedish public health agency stating that 'there were "great risks" that masks would be used incorrectly', and later that 'masks are ineffective and that their use could actually increase the spread of Covid-19'. Indeed, the country's chief epidemiologist, Anders Tegnell, even wrote to the European Centre for Disease Prevention and Control in April 2020 warning against the advice to wear masks because it 'would . . . imply that the spread is airborne, which would seriously harm further communication and trust among the population and health care workers' (cited in Vogel 2020). By August 2020, Walravens and O'Shea continue, 'when mask-wearing was becoming widespread in other European countries, Tegnell said that the evidence for mask-wearing was "astonishingly weak" and that their use could increase the spread of the virus'. Finally, the Swedish prime minister announced a U-turn, mandating the use of masks on public transport only, and with a confusing set of rules: masks were to be worn on public transport 'from 7am to 9am and 4pm to 6pm, for those born "in 2004 and before" who do not have a reserved seat'. Predictably, only 50% of commuters complied. As Walravens and O'Shea conclude, 'the public transport announcement was not only confusing due to its complexity but also due to the fact that its content directly contradicts the mask guidance from March until December'.

Because no story exists in a vacuum but must be situated within wider narratives to be understood and assessed, a high level of structural coherence is not sufficient for the audience to decide whether to adhere to a given narrative. 'The meaning and merit of a story', Fisher explains, 'are always a matter of how it stands with or against other stories' (Fisher 1997:316). The second component of narrative probability, material coherence, therefore concerns how a narrative relates to other (potentially competing) narratives on the same issue that we are familiar with and willing to entertain. It is partly by appeal to material coherence, by 'juxtaposing stories that purport to tell the "truth" about a given matter', that we are able to 'discern factual errors, omission of important arguments, and other sorts of distortion' (Fisher 1994:24). Arguments both for and against measures such as lockdowns and the closing or opening of schools during the Covid-19 crisis rely heavily on charges of material incoherence to discredit the opposing camp and win adherents.

Describing himself as 'no lockdown junkie' nor 'a wobbly-lipped pantry boy who's scared of a bit of flu', Christopher Snowdon, head of Lifestyle Economics at the Institute of Economic Affairs, defends the third national lockdown announced in England as follows in an article published in *Quillette* on 16 January 2021 (Snowdon 2021):

> I had hoped that we could muddle through with local restrictions, but the emergence in December of an extraordinarily infectious new strain put an end to that. The number of COVID cases doubled in the first half of December and doubled again in the second half. Much of London, Kent, and Essex seemed impervious to even the stringent tier 4 restrictions. We did not need a model from Imperial College to see which way this was going. In London and the south-east, there are now more people in hospital with COVID-19 than at the peak of the first wave. There are more on ventilators too, despite doctors using mechanical ventilation less than they did in the spring. It is going to get worse for some time to come. We had to get the numbers down.

The 'facts' cited in the above stretch (for instance, that a new extraordinarily infectious strain had emerged in December, or that there are now more people hospitalized in London than at the peak of the first wave), and many others used in the article to make the case for the necessity of the latest lockdown are drawn from other narratives in circulation at the time and judged to be relevant to the issue at hand. They are facts insofar as Snowdon subscribes to the narratives from which they are drawn.

In 'The case against lockdown: a reply to Christopher Snowdon', also published in *Quillette* on 5 February 2021, Toby Young, editor of *Lockdownsceptics.com*, likewise details various 'facts' derived from narratives similarly in circulation at the time and to which he subscribes in order to point to material incoherence in Snowdon's account (Young 2021):

> If lockdowns work, you'd expect to see an inverse correlation between the severity of the NPIs [non-pharmaceutical interventions] a country puts in place and the number of COVID deaths per capita, but you don't. On the contrary, deaths per million were actually lower in those US states that didn't shut down than in those that did – at least in the first seven-and-a-half months of last year. Trying to explain away these inconvenient facts by factoring in any

number of variables – average age, hours of sunlight, population density – doesn't seem to help. There's no signal in that noise.

Incidentally, Snowdon's claim that the first British lockdown reduced COVID infections is easy to debunk. You just look at when deaths peaked in England and Wales – April 8th – go back three weeks, which is the estimated time from infection to death among the roughly one in 400 infected people who succumb to the disease, and you get to March 19th, indicating infections peaked five days before the lockdown was imposed. Even Chris Whitty, England's Chief Medical Officer, acknowledged that the reproduction rate was falling before the first hammer came down.

Among other pieces of information derived from a variety of sources, Young accepts as fact that 'deaths per million were actually lower in those US states that didn't shut down than in those that did' and considers this as a competing narrative that has relevance to the issue at hand and that Snowdon has chosen not to bring into the argument.

Similarly, when the well-known Italian philosopher Giorgio Agamben initiated a heated debate in February 2020 following publication of a blog post titled 'The invention of a pandemic',[4] many of the arguments against his rejection of what he described as 'frenetic, irrational and entirely unfounded emergency measures adopted against an alleged epidemic of coronavirus' centred on instances of material incoherence. Citing the National Research Council in Italy as his source for asserting that Covid-19 is not much different from the flu and hence does not warrant the drastic measures being introduced by government, Agamben argued that

> The disproportionate reaction to what according to the CNR [Consiglio Nazionale delle Ricerche] is something not too different from the normal flus that affect us every year is quite blatant. It is almost as if with terrorism exhausted as a cause for exceptional measures, the invention of an epidemic offered the ideal pretext for scaling them up beyond any limitation.

In one of the many responses that followed, both supportive and dismissive, Jean-Luc Nancy begins with what he presents as two instances of material incoherence in Agamben's narrative:

> Giorgio Agamben, an old friend, argues that the coronavirus is hardly different from a normal flu. He forgets that for the 'normal' flu there is a vaccine that has been proven effective. And even that needs to be readapted to viral mutations year after year. Despite this, the 'normal' flu always kills several people, while coronavirus, against which there is no vaccine, is evidently capable of causing far higher levels of mortality. The difference (according to sources of the same type as those Agamben uses) is about 1 to 30: it does not seem an insignificant difference to me.

The availability of a flu vaccine and lack of it in the case of Covid-19 is a piece of information deemed relevant to the narrative woven by Agamben but not brought to the attention of the reader. As is the 'fact', drawn from the same source used by Agamben according to Nancy, that the difference between the flu and Covid-19 in terms of fatality is 1 to 30. These missing elements of the narrative provide a basis for considering Agamben's story of what is happening in the context of the pandemic unreliable.

---

[4] See www.journal-psychoanalysis.eu/coronavirus-and-philosophers/ (Agamben's article is published in Italian on Quodlibet, www.quodlibet.it/giorgio-agamben-l-invenzione-di-un-epidemia).

Before we discuss the third component of narrative probability or coherence, namely characterological coherence, it has to be acknowledged that the distinction between structural and material coherence is far from clear cut. While it implies a clear boundary between the components of distinct narratives (those within the text or narrative being assessed and others that are recovered from external sources), this boundary is ultimately constructed by those elaborating an argument and may or may not be accepted by the auditors. For instance, the narrative of a new strain of the virus emerging in the UK in December 2020 is woven by Snowdon into the overall narrative of lockdowns now being necessary and lends structural coherence to his story. It is totally ignored by Young in his rebuttal, implying that it lies outside the scope of the narrative he is contesting. As Baker (2006:148) thus argues:

> The overlap between structural and material coherence is a by-product of two assumptions ... First, narratives construct reality for us; they do not represent it. This means that any boundaries assumed to exist between separate narratives are constructed by us in the course of elaborating the narratives in question; they are not stable, solid boundaries that we simply have to 'discover' and can easily agree on. Second, narratives are not tied to individual, concrete texts but are usually diffuse and have to be pieced together from a variety of sources. Our assessment of the integrity of a diffuse narrative – such as 'America spreading democracy and dignity abroad' – may invoke structural or material coherence, depending on how we piece the narrative together and what we construct as lying within or outside its boundaries.

Beyond structural and material coherence, Fisher (1987:47) argues that 'coherence in life and literature requires that characters behave characteristically'; indeed, without the kind of predictability that arises from characters behaving consistently there can be 'no trust, no community, no rational human order' (Fisher 1987:47). Characterological coherence, the third component of narrative probability, is assessed on the basis of the perceived reliability of the character(s) associated with the story – both narrator(s) and actor(s) depicted or appealed to in the narrative. It is routinely signalled by the familiar practice of citation and references in academic and scientific writing (Baker 2006:149). Above all, however, it is assessed on the basis of the 'intelligence, integrity and goodwill (ethos) of the author, the values she or he embodies and would advance in the world' (Fisher 1994:24).

The story of Neil Ferguson, the Imperial College epidemiologist whose modelling of the virus is thought to have played a major role in persuading the British government to press ahead with a full national lockdown on 23 March 2020, rather than follow the Swedish model, is a case in point. Ferguson could be regarded as the 'narrator' or 'author' of a widely circulated and influential narrative in support of a strict lockdown policy. Although he later insisted that 'his university department's role and his in particular have been overstated', *The Guardian*, among many other sources, insists 'there's little doubt that he became the public figurehead for the argument that without a lockdown hundreds of thousands would die in Britain' (Anthony 2020). Depending on what source is consulted to piece together the story of the events that led to his resignation from the government's Scientific Advisory Group for Emergencies (SAGE) in May 2020, we may reach different assessments of the extent to which he exhibited characterological (in)coherence when his own behaviour was found to be at odds with his official advice. Some sources (narrators of competing narratives of the event) led with headlines such as 'Government scientist Neil Ferguson resigns after breaking lockdown rules to meet his married lover: Prof Ferguson allowed the woman to visit him at home during the lockdown while lecturing the public on the need for strict social distancing' (*The Daily Telegraph*, 5 May 2020).[5] The *Telegraph* article goes on to quote Sir Iain Duncan Smith, the former leader of the Conservative party, as saying: 'Scientists like him have told us we should not be doing it, so surely in his case it is a case of we have been doing as he says and he has been doing as he wants to'. *The Independent* headline on the same day read: 'Neil Ferguson: Government coronavirus adviser quits after home visit from married lover' (Cowburn 2020). *The Independent* went on to report details that are clearly considered pertinent to assessing the extent of Neil Ferguson's characterological (in)coherence:

> It was claimed that Prof Ferguson allowed a woman – described as his 'lover' – to visit him at home in London on at least two occasions during the lockdown despite strict rules against mixing households. The woman reportedly lives with her husband and children.
>
> . . .
>
> The day after the lockdown was announced, on 24 March, Dr Jenny Harries, the deputy chief medical officer, said that couples who do not cohabit must either move in together or not meet at all for the duration of the restrictive measures.
>
> The woman who visited Prof Ferguson is said to have entered his home on 30 March and 8 April.

This type of detail – including the status of Ferguson's lover as married with children and the fact that the rules were broken twice rather than once against clearly worded advice from the deputy chief medical officer – is important in painting a negative picture of the character under scrutiny. Such details undermine the coherence of Ferguson as a character whose advice may provide a warrant for adherence to the narrative supporting a full national lockdown.

Other details missing from *The Daily Telegraph* and *The Independent* stories were reported by *The Guardian* on the same day and are likely to have mitigated the perception of characterological incoherence for some parts of the audience to some extent. Acknowledging merely that Ferguson flouted the rules 'by receiving visits from his lover at his home' and that the visits 'clearly contravene the government's "stay at home, save lives" message, which urges people to remain within their family groups and not mix with members of other households', *The Guardian*'s report quotes Ferguson's reference to the incident as 'an error of judgement' (Stewart 2020). It then goes on to paint a very positive picture of his character:

> Colleagues have described Ferguson, 51 – whose background is in modelling rather than medicine – as a workaholic.
>
> His colleague Christl Donnelly told the Guardian earlier this year: 'He works harder than anyone I have ever met. He is simultaneously attending very large numbers of meetings while running the group from an organisational point of view and doing programming himself. Any one of those things could take somebody their full time.
>
> 'One of his friends said he should slow down – this is a marathon not a sprint. He said he is going to do the marathon at sprint speed. It is not just work ethic – it is also energy. He seems to be able to keep going. He must sleep a bit, but I think not much'.

Not only do narratives that impact our assessment of characterological coherence vary depending on who is narrating and what stakes they have in portraying a given

---

character from a specific light; they also vary over time. Revisiting the issue in December 2020, *The Guardian* featured an interview with Neil Ferguson in which he provided a wider context for his 'error of judgement' (Anthony 2020). Back in the first half of 2020, we are told,

> he was putting in 16- to 18-hour shifts until, as he puts it, he had 'a kind of week off in May'. He's referring to the exposure of an incident in which his lover left her family home and visited him on at least two occasions, thus breaking lockdown rules. Some sections of the press could barely conceal their jubilation.
>
> . . . .
>
> He says that negative attention predated the quarantine transgression. 'People had set up bots, which bombarded my email account with over a million emails a day from late March onwards', he explains.
>
> He was also the subject of countless hacking attempts and a torrent of 'very unpleasant messages'. He found the sheer weight of the aggression 'emotionally debilitating'.

This type of contextual detail that Ferguson is allowed to provide several months after the events that led to his resignation makes it possible for many members of the audience to look back on the entire affair and sympathize with his predicament, excuse his 'error of judgement' on this one occasion. Like Ferguson, many will have been tempted to visit a loved one surreptitiously at some point during the lockdown, but perhaps were fortunate not to be caught and not to be in the public eye and suffer the consequences. If Ferguson, in addition to the pressure and anxiety most people suffered during that period, was also working 16–18 hours a day and battling with such intense hate campaigns, there may be enough warrants for many to (re)assess him as a reliable, trustworthy character and hence to consider his advice on lockdown and other issues as credible after all.

Addressing a wider issue, an open letter[6] signed by 26 scientists – described in a *Nature*'s news roundup[7] on 13 May 2020 as having 'rallied behind' Ferguson – argued that advice provided to the government is not the result of an individual effort but of collaborative work and consensus among researchers. The signatories do not question the fact that Ferguson's apparent lack of integrity discredited his advice. Rather they argue that the real narrator of the lockdown story was not Ferguson alone but a whole community of scientists whose 'character' warrants adherence:

> his individual error of judgement has been used to try to discredit the wider scientific basis for the lockdown. This amplifies the misconception that a single scientist was the 'architect of the lockdown', having single-handedly convinced the government to introduce drastic social distancing measures. But while Prof Ferguson is undoubtedly an influential scientist, the reality of how science has informed, and keeps informing decision-making is quite different.

For those to whom this narrative rang true, the need to observe lockdown rules remained part of a credible story that warrants adherence, and the characterological coherence of the (collaborative) narrator was reconstituted.

---

[6] https://docs.google.com/document/u/1/d/e/2PACX-1vSxP91cr4TOPVi9gwW4mGL9BL2wyQAVj FOw-pB2aRe3uXXXIfyDrJpef5Qp0B8_l9en6buM0LTjRSYq/pub.

[7] www.nature.com/articles/d41586-020-01362-0.

Interestingly, another high-profile UK character who was accused by some of a similar breach of lockdown rules, this time in December 2020, received a very different treatment from the media and the public. Captain Sir Tom Moore, affectionately known as Captain Tom (Figure 2.1), was 99 years old and recovering from a broken hip when he decided in April 2020 to raise funds for the National Health Service (NHS) by walking laps in his garden. Starting with a modest goal of £1,000, his story touched the pulse of a nation struggling to come to terms with the reality of the pandemic, and within 24 days he had raised a staggering £33 million, made many media appearances and become a household name. He died in early February 2021, having been knighted by the Queen and honoured in a variety of ways and venues. Given this background and level of visibility, attacks on his character for a similar breach as Ferguson's were vociferously rejected by the mainstream media and seemed to make no difference to the public's trust in him. The story goes as follows. British Airways and Visit Barbados treated Captain Tom and his family to a holiday in Barbados on the occasion of his 100th birthday, in early December 2020, as a reward for his remarkable achievement. Reporting his death from Covid-19 on 3 February 2021, *The Express* was careful to state that he and his family 'set off [on the trip to Barbados] before his hometown of Bedford was placed into Tier 3 on December 19, and later Tier 4 on December 20' (Hawker 2021). Questions could still be asked, of course, about his exposure to the virus during his trip and whether he brought it back to his hometown. *The Express* indirectly refutes this potential charge,

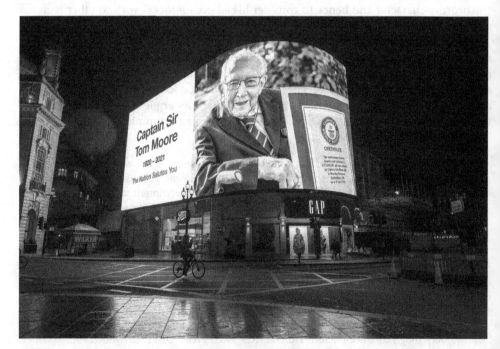

Figure 2.1 A birthday message for Moore was displayed on advertising boards in a deserted Piccadilly Circus in London on April 30 last year. Copyright Chris J Ratcliffe / Stringer / Getty images.

without actually stating it, and goes on to detail some of the many tributes paid to him by leading figures:

> This afternoon, Captain Tom's family released information which revealed he tested positive for coronavirus on January 22 after returning home from hospital where he was diagnosed with pneumonia.
> The family added he was tested regularly for the virus between December 9 and January 12 and each test returned a negative result . . .
> The Prime Minister and the Queen have led the tributes which have poured in from around the world.
> Boris Johnson said: 'Captain Sir Tom Moore was a hero in the truest sense of the word.
> 'In the dark days of the Second World War, he fought for freedom and in the face of this country's deepest post-war crisis, he united us all, he cheered us all up, and he embodied the triumph of the human spirit'.

Some attacks on Captain Tom's character nevertheless followed, but were met with outrage rather than a questioning of his credibility. The British celebrities magazine *Hello*, for instance, reported on 3 February 2021 that Piers Morgan, a high-profile broadcaster and television personality, 'hit out at critics of the holiday – which occurred before strict travel restrictions came into force – and revealed the full extent to which their comments have hurt Sir Tom's loved ones' (Strong 2021). Instead of contesting Captain Tom's behaviour, Morgan berated those who commented negatively on the trip, casting doubt on their integrity rather than his:

> 'I hope you can live with yourselves. I really do, because it was despicable and the very worst of this country is some of the stuff that I read on Twitter and social media in the last few days.
> He continued: 'The Prime Minister rightly came out and condemned it. We have to do something about this. That people think it's ok to abuse the likes of Captain Tom and his family after they raised £39 million for this country, for the NHS'.

Why do charges of characterological incoherence receive such different responses from various groups in society? Perhaps because some characters, like Captain Tom, 'stand in as metaphors for larger ideas and values' (Stache 2018:576); they become larger than life, a character in a story about the nation or about humanity at large, a symbol of generosity of spirit, resilience and other qualities that inspire us and that we particularly need to believe in during a crisis. Questioning the credibility of such characters means questioning more than a piece of advice or account of a set of events: it means questioning values that the audience has invested in emotionally and needs to hold on to at a time of calamity. This may also explain why certain 'facts' like the implications of Captain Tom's trip to Barbados for the spread of Covid-19 in the UK are considered irrelevant to the structural and material coherence of his narrative.

Ultimately, as Fisher (1987:24) explains, despite the components of narrative probability appearing to be identical to formal methods of testing the quality of reasoning of a given message, in each of them 'values are manifest', and at any rate, 'values inform "reason"' (Fisher 1987:24), as will become clearer in our discussion of narrative fidelity.

2.3.2 Narrative Fidelity

Whereas narrative probability concerns 'the formal features of a story conceived as a discrete sequence of thought' (Fisher 1987:88), narrative fidelity 'pertains to the individuated components of stories – whether they represent accurate assertions about social reality and thereby constitute good reasons for belief or action' (Fisher 1987:105). It concerns the truth qualities of a story, that is to say, how well the narrated experiences resonate with those of readers and thus appear as 'real' (authentic) experiences. This means that assessing a narrative for fidelity proceeds by examining the components of the logic of good reasons, which allow us to 'weigh values in discourse to determine their worthiness as a basis of belief and action' (Fisher 1994:24). According to Fisher, the components of the **logic of good reasons** correspond with the five steps that characterize the **logic of reasons**, which he summarizes as follows (Fisher 1987:109):

> First one considers whether the statements in a message that purport to be 'facts' are indeed 'facts' ... Second, one tries to determine whether those that have been offered are in any way distorted or taken out of context. Third, one recognizes and assesses the various patterns of reasoning, using mainly standards from informal logic. Fourth, one assesses the relevance of individual arguments to the decision the message concerns, not only are these arguments sound, but are they also all the arguments that should be considered in the case. Fifth ... one makes a judgement as to whether or not the message directly addresses the 'real' issue in the case. The components needed to transform the logic of reason into a logic of good reason are also fivefold.

Using similar criteria to those of the logic of reasons, Baker (2006:152–153) explains the logic of good reasons as follows:

- *Fact.* We begin our assessment of fidelity by asking what implicit and explicit values are embedded in a narrative. This criterion assumes that the narrative itself is a story of values, and that we can trace and identify these values in the narrative.
- *Relevance.* Like the second component of the logic of reasons, this criterion concerns the relevance of what is presented in the narrative; but the focus here is on values rather than arguments and facts: 'Are the values appropriate to the nature of the decision that the message bears upon?' Included in this question must be concern for omitted, distorted and misrepresented values.
- *Consequence.* This criterion focuses on the real world consequences of accepting the values elaborated in the narrative. Here, we ask '[w]hat would be the effects of adhering to the values – for one's concept of oneself, for one's behavior, for one's relationships with others and society, and to the process of rhetorical transaction?'.
- *Consistency.* 'Are the values confirmed or validated in one's personal experience, in the lives or statements of others whom one admires and respects, and in a conception of the best audience that one can conceive?'. This is a question of whether the values expressed in the narrative are consistent with one's own experience of the world.
- *Transcendent issue or values.* This is the most important component of the logic of good reasons and hence the most important criterion in assessing any narrative. Under this heading, Fisher invites us to ask whether 'the values the message offers ... constitute the ideal basis for human conduct', irrespective of the facts and '[e]ven if a prima-facie case exists or a burden of proof has been established' in relation to a specific narrative. Fisher stresses that identifying and assessing the transcendent value in a narrative 'is clearly the paramount issue that confronts those responsible for decisions that impinge on the nature, the quality, and the continued existence of human life, especially in such fields as biology and weapons technology and employment'.

As evident from the above summary, narrative fidelity ultimately rests on an assessment of transcendental values, as we saw earlier in the example of Siegel's (2017) review of Richard Herrnstein and Charles Murray's *The Bell Curve*. Transcendental values are rarely the subject of dispute and are often taken for granted, but 'when brought to the surface they reveal one's most fundamental commitments' (Fisher 1987:109). Transcendental values often exceed everyday values such as precision, accuracy, accord with existing knowledge, truthfulness and usefulness in the context of scholarly work. They may also exceed pragmatic values such as efficiency and success. The ultimate values we live by 'look not only to the past and present, but also to the future, the future beyond the immediate moment'; they include 'justice, happiness, and humanity', but for Fisher the ultimate value is 'love, that is an abiding concern for the welfare and well-being of others' (Fisher 1994:28).

Different sets of transcendental values may come into conflict and lead to major public controversies, especially during prolonged crises such as pandemics. It is also during such crises that narrators are more likely to spell out what they see as ultimate, non-negotiable values that must be protected at all costs, whereas in normal circumstances such values are usually left implicit and taken for granted rather than explicitly articulated. Two examples will suffice to demonstrate the kind of tension that drives different people to accept or reject a narrative on the basis of such values, however well supported the narrative may be, logically and scientifically.

Toby Young's rebuttal of Christopher Snowdon's argument in favour of the third UK lockdown in January 2021 (discussed under material coherence earlier) attracted many comments. One commentator makes explicit what he or she considers to be a transcendent, non-negotiable value that trumps all other values (Snowdon 2021):

> But I've recently realised my own prejudices are clouding my judgment. I'm desperately trying to find an angle to win the argument against lockdowns, a key indicator that proves I'm right. But what for?
> This is the thing, more so than anything on Toby's website, or explained in Ivor Cummins stats, or Mike Yeadon's science, I've realised that the numbers aren't the key to my argument. My argument, my opinion and my belief is much more simple and incontestable than any figures. Simply put, enforced lockdowns are wrong, amoral, evil and not an option. No matter the cases, deaths, NHS pressure ... it's never acceptable to restrict the liberty of millions of people to meet, talk, play, work, sing, learn or worship. Under any circumstances. The virus occurred naturally and deaths from it are very sad. But the imposition on liberty and the damage caused by lockdowns is wilfully inflicted, unacceptable and unforgivable.

The value that this particular commentator sees as sacrosanct is freedom and individual liberty. Others writing in a variety of venues during that period expressed commitments to a very different set of values.

Many arguments against lockdown, apart from those which assume that the pandemic is a manufactured hoax, generally accept that without a lockdown there would be higher fatalities, mostly among the elderly and those with underlying health conditions. Writing for *The Guardian* on 30 May 2020, as lockdown rules were increasingly being relaxed in the UK, a palliative care doctor offers a visceral, heartfelt account of what it was like to work with Covid-19 patients. Headed '"This man knows he's dying as surely as I do": a doctor's dispatches from the NHS frontline' (Clarke 2020), much of her narrative revolves around a particular patient she is about to attend to, Winston, who is on the verge of dying and whose life and humanity, she argues, are obscured by the 'mathematical abstraction' of modelling and statistics. 'Here in the hospital', she points out, 'the pandemic is a matter of flesh and blood. It unfolds one human being at a time'.

Winston is an 89-year-old man from a care home who 'used to work in the local glass factory. His wife died three years ago. He has two sons called Michael and Robert'. As the story unfolds, Dr Clarke adds details that highlight not only the humanity of Winston and his two sons who are watching him die, but also the brutalizing inhumanity to which healthcare providers like herself are subjected by the pandemic:

> I'm already wearing my mask. I've pressed the metal strip down hard on to my nose and cheekbones, endeavouring to make it airtight. Now I layer on more protection. Apron, gloves and visor, the minimum with which we approach our patients these days.
>
> In PPE [personal protective equipment], everything is sticky and stifling. Voices are muffled and smiles obscured. Sweat starts trickling into your underwear. Even breathing takes more effort. Behind our masks, we strain to hear each other speak and are forced to second guess our colleagues' expressions. Being protected entails being dehumanised.
>
> . . . My hospital badge is hidden from view and my eyes – the only part of my face still visible – are obscured by a layer of Perspex. So much for the healing presence of the bedside physician. I scarcely look human.
>
> All those arcs and sweeps and projections and opinions – the endless, esoteric, disorientating debates about whether flattening or crushing the curve is more desirable – arrive, in the end, at precisely this point, this moment of cold simplicity. Six feet away, a father, a man I am yet to lay eyes on, is dying of a disease only named a month ago. . . .
>
> Everything about this is wrong. The physical barriers between us. The harsh and jarring words that conceal rising panic. The glaring need – that can't be met – to rip off the masks and gloves and shake hands, sit down, read each other's expressions and begin, inch by inch, to cross the gulf that divides us.

This narrative evokes transcendental values with which many readers will identify: compassion, respect for human dignity and the sanctity of life. Rather than engaging in 'reasoned' arguments about the merits or otherwise of lockdowns or herd immunity, Dr Clarke appeals to our shared humanity. The values which inform her decisions – and, she hopes, those of her readers – are spelled out unequivocally in the concluding paragraphs, and contrasted with other values (such as economic productivity and individual freedom) that feature in many of the debates around Covid-19:

> You could argue – indeed, some commentators have essentially done so – that there was little point to a man like Winston. He was 89 years old, after all, and probably hadn't been economically productive for three decades. He was lucky, frankly, to have had an innings like that. Of course the young must come first. You might even champion another old man's exploits – the charm and determination and ebullience of Captain Tom – while being secretly at peace with the expendability of certain parts of the herd.
>
> But to those of us up close with this dreadful disease – who see, as we do, the way it suffocates the life from you – such judgments are grotesque. The moment we rank life according to who most 'deserves' it, we have crossed into a realm I don't want to be a part of – and I struggle to believe many other Britons do either. The way out of this pandemic cannot, surely, entail the sacrifice of those deemed less worth saving? . . .
>
> Winston, though vulnerable, was loved and cherished. His death was not inevitable, his time hadn't come. He was no more disposable than any of us.

Narratives such as Dr Clarke's, which espouse values of humanity and compassion, ring true for many but by no means all members of society. Large sectors of every society continue to argue against lockdowns, for herd immunity, and believe that sacrificing men like Winston to allow the majority of productive, healthy citizens to live their lives and keep the economy going is regrettable but inevitable. This argument also appeals to transcendent values: those of expediency, material success and political acumen. As Fisher (1987:188; emphasis in original) explains, people who rank these values higher than all others have found them '*relevant* to their material lives, *consequential* in determining their survival and well-being, *consistent* with statements made by those who subscribe to the myth that humans are masters of their fates and with examples of those who succeeded by following it'. These are 'realistic' values that appeal to many, but Fisher suggests that idealistic stories such as Dr Clarke's will always resonate with large sectors of the public. These stories 'generate adherence because they are coherent and "ring true" to life *as we would like to live it*'. Their appeal 'resides in their evoking the best in people and activating it' (Fisher 1987:187; emphasis in original).

Fisher's narrative paradigm is not without its critics and limitations, and we will return to this issue in the final chapter to acknowledge the most important of these limitations and suggest some ways in which the model's weaknesses might be addressed. Warnick (1987), for example, has argued that Fisher's theory is based on a simplified understanding of the rational logic that he (Fisher) refutes. She claims that Fisher only attacks one subform of what he calls traditional rationality – technical rationality – without acknowledging other forms, such as practical reasoning and moral judgement. Furthermore, while acknowledging that people can be wrong, Fisher is silent on how they can avoid being deluded, given his dismissal of traditional rationality (Warnick 1987:177). As she puts it, 'a rhetorical narrative may "ring true" in the lives of particular audience members, may resonate with their own experience and that of those who they admire, and nevertheless be a bad story' (Warnick 1987:179). Acknowledging this criticism, we do not suggest that everything that 'rings true' to an audience is necessarily good according to some universal standard. We only claim that any argument inevitably adheres to a concept of the good and that to identify and understand this notion is relevant when engaging with or arguing against a particular position.

We revisit the narrative paradigm and attempt to expand and update it Chapter 6. The next three chapters, meanwhile, examine different perspectives on some of the major controversies surrounding Covid-19, using the logic of good reasons to interrogate the values that inform various positions and the consequences of adhering to them.

Whose Evidence? What Rationality? The Face Mask Controversy

Arguments about the pros and cons and possible effectiveness of face masks during the Covid-19 crisis have occupied considerable space in specialist, medical venues such as peer-reviewed journals and science blogs, as well as public forums such as mainstream media and social media – the latter attracting contributions from medical specialists and lay members of the public alike. The debate has often been heated, and there have been reports of individuals resisting the stipulation to wear face masks in shops and on airplanes, at times leading to acts of physical violence. Drawing on the narrative paradigm, this chapter examines some of the arguments for and against face masks as articulated by a diverse range of individuals and constituencies within and beyond the Anglophone and European world, the justifications given in each case, and their underlying values and logics.

At the heart of the controversy surrounding the stipulation to wear face masks during the Covid-19 pandemic is an institutional narrative that has been characterized by conspicuous structural and material incoherence from the very start. The medical community and World Health Organization (WHO) both gave conflicting messages about the benefits and safety of using face masks throughout. In turn, as Austin Wright argues in the October 2020 issue of *UChicago News*, the uncertainty created by expert mixed messaging allowed politicians such as Donald Trump and their advocates 'to create competing politicized narratives that weaken[ed] public compliance' (A. Wright 2020). These competing narratives often appealed to nationalistic, misogynist and homophobic tropes that tend to resonate among sizeable sections of the population during periods of extreme insecurity, including wars and pandemics, when people feel the need to reaffirm threatened social identities. Disagreements among members of the medical community and weak or conflicting recommendations on the part of organizations such as WHO and US Centers for Disease Control and Prevention thus created a space for the UK's Boris Johnson, Brazil's Jair Bolsonaro and other high-profile personalities to amplify values such as masculinity and personal liberty at the expense of public safety and social responsibility. We explore the extent to which the narrative paradigm can explain this trajectory, and further enrich it with the concepts of narrative accrual and identification where relevant to offer a more cogent account of some of the extreme responses to face masking that we have witnessed in the context of Covid-19.

3.1 Structural and Material (In)coherence in Expert Narratives

Conflicting messages about face masks issued by health authorities and members of the medical community, particularly during the early days of the pandemic, were informed by divergent understandings of the transmission route of the virus. There is general consensus among experts that virus transmission either occurs directly (between persons) or indirectly (through objects). Object contamination as well as contamination of persons at a short distance happen through large droplets while airborne transmission via aerosols can occur over an extended distance through the respiratory tract (Zhang et al. 2020). With regards to public health measures, transmission through contact and droplets is typically controlled through physical distancing, hand washing, surface cleansing and wearing masks if people stand less than 6 feet apart, while the measures to control airborne diseases include ventilation and wearing face coverings when sharing air (Czypionk et al. 2020). Nevertheless, advice issued by health authorities at different times has reflected structural incoherence in terms of both the recommendations and their theoretical underpinnings.

The WHO gradually moved towards recommending face masks in every situation, while the theory supporting the recommendations was only partly modified accordingly. In April 2020, the WHO's advice was to reserve the use of masks for health personnel, arguing that 'there is currently no evidence that wearing a mask (whether medical or other types) by healthy persons in the wider community setting, including universal community masking, can prevent them from infection with respiratory viruses, including COVID-19' (WHO 2020a). The UK's Chief Medical Officer, Jonathan Van Tam, reiterated the same message at a Downing Street Press Conference on 3 April (Schofield 2020):

> I was on the phone this morning to a colleague in Hong Kong whose [sic] done the evidence review for the World Health Organisation on face masks.
> We are of the same mind that there is no evidence that the general wearing of face masks by the public who are well affects the spread of the disease in our society.
> Yes it is true that we do see very large amounts of mask-wearing in south-east Asia, but we have always seen that for many decades.
> In terms of the hard evidence, we do not recommend face masks for general wearing for the public.

The WHO went on to even warn against the use of masks in community settings on the basis that it runs the risk of creating a false sense of security and poses a possible risk of self-contamination. It further argued that 'the two main routes of transmission of the Covid-19 virus are respiratory droplets and contact' and denounced the claim that Covid-19 is airborne as 'misinformation' and 'incorrect' (Figure 3.1).[1] On 5 June 2020, the organization updated its advice, this time encouraging the general public to wear masks in specific situations and settings where physical distancing could not be achieved. The main route to transmission was still considered to be droplets and contact. However, the guidelines also now acknowledged that 'in specific circumstances and settings in which procedures that generate aerosols are performed, airborne transmission of the COVID-19 virus may be possible' but that more research was needed (WHO 2020b). On 1 December 2020, the WHO revised its guidelines again (WHO 2020c). This time it also recommended the use of face coverings in indoor settings where ventilation is poor. Aerosol transmission – described earlier as 'misinformation' – was now clearly implied to be a relevant factor in the spread of the virus. Without acceptance of this theory, the new recommendation would lack structural coherence. This is partly acknowledged, at least as a possible explanation: 'Outside of medical facilities, in addition to droplet and fomite transmission, aerosol transmission can occur in specific settings and circumstances, particularly in indoor, crowded and

---

[1] https://twitter.com/WHO/status/1243972193169616898.

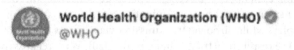

World Health Organization (WHO) ✓
@WHO

···

FACT: #COVID19 is NOT airborne.

The #coronavirus is mainly transmitted through droplets generated when an infected person coughs, sneezes or speaks.

To protect yourself:
-keep 1m distance from others
-disinfect surfaces frequently
-wash/rub your 🖐
-avoid touching your 👀 👃 👄

FACT CHECK: COVID-19 is NOT airborne

The virus that causes COVID-19 is mainly transmitted through droplets generated when an infected person coughs, sneezes, or speaks. These droplets are too heavy to hang in the air. They quickly fall on floors or surfaces.

You can be infected by breathing in the virus if you are within 1 metre of a person who has COVID-19, or by touching a contaminated surface and then touching your eyes, nose or mouth before washing your hands.

To protect yourself, keep at least 1 metre distance from others and disinfect surfaces that are touched frequently. Regularly clean your hands thoroughly and avoid touching your eyes, mouth, and nose.

March 28 2020

#coronavirus #COVID19

Figure 3.1 WHO Fact Check tweeted 29 March 2020

inadequately ventilated spaces, where infected persons spend long periods of time with others' (WHO 2020c). However, 'high quality research' is said to be required and the overarching theory is still that 'SARS-CoV-2 *mainly* spreads between people when an infected person is in close contact with another person' (our emphasis). Despite the change of advice, the WHO claimed that 'there is only limited and inconsistent scientific evidence to support the effectiveness of masking of healthy people in the community' (WHO 2020c).

Within the space of nine months, advice issued by the WHO had thus changed from warning against the risk of community masking to encouraging its use. Meanwhile, the theoretical underpinning of the advice had shifted from denouncing airborne transmission as misinformation to including it as evidence, albeit reluctantly. Importantly, at no time did the WHO publicly correct its earlier statements and at the time of writing has not deleted its tweets and fact sheets supporting its original take on the issue of face masking. Its warnings against spreading 'misinformation' about aerosol transmission still appear on several platforms alongside its new recommendations, which are informed by the same theory it had previously rejected. In a debate with aerosol scientists on 9 April 2021, Professor John Conly, who is part of the WHO's group of experts advising on coronavirus guidelines, admitted that there might be 'situational' airborne transmission but that he would still 'like to see a much higher level of scientific evidence'.[2] However, he did not offer any explanation of what 'situational' means in this respect and whether it refers to any indoor situation, in which case, as noted in one of the numerous tweets commenting on the debate, 'that's kind of a common situation'.[3]

National guidance on the use of face masks has also changed during the pandemic and varied significantly between different nations and regions. A number of Asian countries recommended the use of medical masks by the public very early in the pandemic, and this recommendation did not result in any controversies. Goodman (2020) suggests that the high levels of compliance with face masking in Asian countries is due to the fact that 'they never forgot the lessons of the Manchurian plague' in 1910–1911, when bodies piled up on the streets of Harbin and more than 60,000 people lost their lives within the space of four months. This was when a young doctor by the name of Wu Lien first introduced the idea of masking. He 'wrapped the faces of health workers and grave diggers in layers of cotton and gauze to filter out the bacteria, creating the ancestor of the modern N95 respirator mask'. He also urged everyone to cover their faces, having realized that the disease was 'carried through the air, in respiratory droplets from breath' (Goodman 2020). Wu was the first Chinese to win the Nobel Prize and thus remains a source of pride for his compatriots. In narrative paradigm terms, he possesses a very high level of characterological coherence and his scientific legacy remains credible. For Asian populations who had recently lived through the SARS outbreak in 2003, moreover, narratives that emphasize the need to take the pandemic seriously and adopt precautionary measures to protect the population from it also resonate strongly. Goodman (2020) suggests that while face masks were also widely used to control the 1918 flu pandemic, their importance seems to have been forgotten in the West.

Unlike Asian countries, Norway and Sweden continued to restrict their advice to specific situations. In August 2020, Norwegian health authorities recommended the use of face masks on public transport in situations where high levels of transmission are likely and when a physical distance of one meter cannot be maintained, for instance during the rush hour (NIPH 2020a). In October 2020, the Norwegian Institute of Public Health (NIPH) extended the recommendation to all situations where a high level of transmission is likely and where it is difficult to maintain a safe distance. It further emphasized that face masks could be used in addition to but not to replace other measures (NIPH 2020b). Physical distancing and hand hygiene were however considered the 'most important measures to prevent infection', and the primary transmission route is to date believed to be droplet infection. Sweden's policy on face masks has been even more restrictive. As

---

[2] https://ucalgary.yuja.com/V/Video?v=332352&node=1205653&a=385475807&autoplay=1.
[3] https://twitter.com/Miscellaneousmm/status/1380754113063882762?s=20.

mentioned in Chapter 2, the country's chief epidemiologist, Anders Tegnell, explicitly warned against the use of masks because it 'would imply the spread is airborne', which would 'seriously harm further communication and trust' (cited in Vogel 2020). In December 2020, the Swedish government modified its policy and recommended face coverings on public transport for people born in 2004 or earlier, and only on working weekdays between 7:00 and 9:00 and from 16:00 to 18:00.

The incoherence of public health recommendations must be understood against the backdrop of inconsistencies in the scientific discourse throughout the pandemic. Policy recommendations tend to draw heavily on systematic reviews of scientific literature, which summarize and draw conclusions based on the current state of the art. However, many of the systematic reviews on face coverings in the context of Covid-19 reached contradictory conclusions despite being broadly based on the same body of evidence. While Greenhalgh and Howard (2020), for instance, reached a conclusion that strongly supported the use of face masks, Brainard et al. (2020) concluded that 'evidence is not sufficiently strong to support widespread use of facemasks as a protective measure against COVID-19'. As Greenhalgh (2020a) has pointed out in a blog piece on the website of the Centre for Evidence-Based Medicine, the difference between these and other conflicting views seems to arise not from what the evidence *is* but from what it *means*. She emphasizes five areas of contestation in the face-masking controversy which underpin the structural and material incoherence evident in institutional narratives:

- Is the absence of a definitive randomised controlled trial, along with the hypothetical possibility of harm (for example from risk compensation) a good reason to hold back from changing policy? . . .
- Should we take account of stories reported in the lay press, such as those of single individuals apparently responsible for infecting dozens and even hundreds of others at rallies, prayer meetings or choir practices? . . .
- Should we extrapolate from laboratory experiments on the filtration capacity of different fabrics to estimate what is likely to happen when people wear them in real life? . . .
- Should we use anecdotal reports of some people wearing their masks 'wrongly' or intermittently to justify not recommending them to everyone? . . .
- Should we take account of the possibility that promoting masks for the lay public may lead to a shortage of precious personal protective equipment (PPE) for healthcare workers? . . . .

Linked to this discussion is also a debate about how to use the precautionary principle in the context of face masks. The standard approach, which has been defended by some, suggests caution in the uptake of innovations with known benefits but uncertain or unmeasurable downsides, as in the case of the implementation of new pharmaceutical treatments (Martin et al. 2020a). At the start of the Covid-19 pandemic, for instance, John Ioannidis – a specialist in epidemiology, population health and biomedical data science at the Stanford School of Medicine – called attempts to impose what he saw as 'draconian political decisions' such as mandating the use of face coverings in the absence of evidence 'a fiasco in the making' (Cayley 2020). Greenhalgh (2020b), by contrast, has suggested a supplementary approach that advocates precaution in the case of non-intervention when serious harm is already happening and a proposed intervention may reduce that harm. It is worth noting that a systematic review and meta-analysis on the effectiveness of public health measures to reduce the incidence of Covid-19 – specifically, handwashing, face masking and social distancing – published in the *British Medical Journal* (*BMJ*) on 18 November (Talic et al. 2021) reported that face masking led to 'a 53% reduction in covid-19 incidence', but concluded that 'more high level evidence is required to provide unequivocal support for the effectiveness of the universal use of face masks'. Well over a year after the mandate on wearing face masks in public was imposed and then lifted in many countries, the evidence from randomized controlled trials was still not conclusive. The jury remains out on this particular issue at the time of writing, and the controversies and contradictions continue to plague public policy.

More broadly, these conceptual inconsistencies also relate to different understandings of what counts as evidence in a public health context. Evidence-based medicine (EBM) has partly grown out of scepticism about the value of mechanistic reasoning as the foundation for clinical decision making. While the key characteristic of clinical decision making prior to the emergence of EBM was reliance on knowledge of mechanisms in the human body to make predictions about the outcomes of interventions, EBM reasoning relies on treatment recommendations distilled from experimental studies of interventions, for which no mechanistic justification may be known (Andersen 2012). This partly explains why some EBM proponents (including health authorities like the WHO) can live with inconsistencies between mask recommendations and their mechanical justifications, although these inconsistencies might be very confusing for people less familiar with the fundamental presuppositions of the relevant scientific paradigm. In public health, however, interventions are most often developed and tested pragmatically and locally. Natural experiments are highly valued and evidence is drawn from a whole range of different sources, including individual experiences of interventions in local settings and basic science research (Greenhalgh 2020b). In the context of the pandemic, we have experienced a clash between these different paradigms of evidence, which in turn has led to incoherence and confusion about the conclusions to be drawn from the scientific evidence. We have also been exposed to the limits of applied science in general in the context of a raging pandemic that does not allow enough time for conflicting scientific studies to be replicated and fine-tuned. As David Kriebel, Professor of Epidemiology at the University of Massachusetts-Lowell, argues, 'science is self-correcting, given enough time. But currently there is not enough time for science to self-correct when it's being used to craft public health policy'. His advice is that rather than 'clamoring for scientific studies to back up mandates on mask use', we should seek more transparency in public health messaging and share the uncertainty with the public – tell people honestly: 'Mask use is our best judgment right now, and we will tell you if we get more evidence' (quoted in Soucheray 2020).

The debate about the use of masks in schools has added a new layer of complexity to the epistemic controversies that characterize scientific enquiry. From merely being a debate involving different public health opinions and divergent understandings of what counts as evidence in a public health setting, the various arguments now draw on several other forms of expertise and have become a source from which evidence of material incoherence may be drawn. The answer to whether face masks should be recommended in the school setting largely depends on how the question is framed and which experts are called upon to answer it. Researchers in educational and behavioural science, for instance, have emphasized how wearing masks can affect the ability to communicate and interpret the expressions of teachers and other students and thereby negatively impacts learning and social bonding in the school setting (Spitzer 2020). Some scholars have also claimed that the use of face masks can trigger anxiety and fear among children and even harm their cognitive development (Deoini 2021).

Indeed, public recommendations regarding the use of face masks in schools have been even more confused than the general advice on their use in other settings. In the UK, the prime minister Boris Johnson stated in August 2020 that the idea of school children wearing face masks in classrooms is 'clearly nonsensical': 'You can't teach with face coverings and you can't expect people to learn with face coverings' (Devlin 2020). Yet, in one of the many U-turns that have characterized public policy during the pandemic, he 'bowed to pressure' a few hours later and changed the guidance 'after scores of headteachers broke ranks to urge their use, backed by [the] Labour [Party] and trade unions' (Elgot and Halliday 2020). In March 2021, the Department for Education updated its advice on face coverings following the spread of new, more transmissible variants of the virus. The guidance was now for 'pupils and students in year 7 and above' and their teachers to 'wear face coverings indoors, including classrooms, where social distancing cannot be maintained' (Department of Education 2021). By July 2021, the legal requirement to wear a mask was removed in England, except in hospitals and care homes. In November of the same year, Boris Johnson – the head of the same government that still mandated the use of face masks in healthcare settings – was severely criticized and forced to apologize when he was seen walking without a mask in the corridor in Hexham Hospital, Northumberland (Press Association 2021). Such U-turns and frequent changes in policy have been used as evidence of structural incoherence by the so-called 'Us for them' movement, an anti-mask, grassroots schools campaign backed by thousands of parents and pupils. An open letter to the UK Education Secretary, published on their site, asks for evidence to support the change in policy and points out:[4]

> Last Summer, the Government said masks in classrooms were unnecessary. The Prime Minister described it as 'nonsensical' and said that 'you can't teach with face coverings and you can't expect people to learn with face coverings'. Your own department's August guidance said that they 'can have a negative impact on learning and teaching and so their use in the classroom should be avoided'.

Numerous other challenges to the guidance on wearing face masks in schools rely on pointing out aspects of the structural and/or material incoherence of institutional narratives, within and across different countries. The following two comments on an article published in *The Telegraph* on 26 August 2020 under the title 'We will have a generation of scarred children' demonstrate the challenge to both types of incoherence – structural and material:

> @AJ Boyle
> Face masks send out a message that there's danger, therefore by logic it's not safe for schools to open.
> The teachers that don't want to work now have a point.
> You can't have it both ways Boris, it's either one or the other.

> @Marvin Taylor
> My kids went back to school here in Norway back in May, then a few weeks later had their summer holidays. Now they are back again and things are almost back to normal.
> Not once did they have to wear face masks.

---

[4] https://usforthem.co.uk/open-letters/no-masks-in-class/.

The article itself is interestingly attributed by the newspaper to its readers, rather than to *The Telegraph*,[5] alerting us to the role played by the media in amplifying and sanctioning particular arguments for or against public policies and the values that underpin them.

'We will have a generation of scarred children' – *Telegraph* readers on face masks in schools
Telegraph readers have had their say on face masks in schools
– Headline from a *Telegraph* article

Those for whom a mainstream broadsheet such as *The Telegraph* represents a credible and trustworthy source of information and sober views – in other words, for whom the paper possesses a high level of characterological coherence – will conclude from such coverage that there is a genuine ground swell against the use of face masks in schools, that many parents have real and rational concerns about the dangers associated with them, and will be encouraged to rethink their own take on the issue if it is at odds with this coverage. What is at work in such instances is part of a process of narrative accrual, an important dimension of how narratives evolve and gain adherence over time (Bruner 1991; Baker 2006). Narrative accrual means that repeated exposure to a set of related narratives and their underlying values gradually shapes our outlook on life, and ultimately the transcendental values that inform our judgements and are at the heart of the logic of good reasons, to which we turn next.

3.2 Transcendental Values, Narrative Accrual and Narrative Identification

While some of those who have argued against the use of face masks have expressed their concerns in measured language and explained them with reference to scientific evidence, or lack of it, others have acted in ways that are strongly confrontational, and often violent towards others. From the unmasked protestors in Trafalgar Square who carried signs with slogans such as 'masks are muzzles' and 'Covid is a hoax' (Philipose 2020, in *The Indian Express*), to those who stood outside the Sephora Beverley Hills Beauty Store chanting 'No More Masks' and holding pieces of paper with messages such as 'Sephora Supports Communism' or shouting 'Sephora is agent of Chinese government' (Wittner 2021), behaviour that would normally be seen as bizarre and restricted to a small fringe seems to have become the order of the day during the Covid-19 crisis. The logic of good reasons and the concept of transcendental values allow us to understand some but not all such responses to face masking, for as McClure (2009:205) explains, the problem with the concept of fidelity is that 'belief in a story is accounted for by the fact that it's already believed without ever having to explain why it's believed in the first instance'. In what follows, we draw on Bruner (1991) and McClure (2009) where necessary to address this weakness in Fisher's model and make sense of some of the beliefs and behaviour that appear resistant to explanation in terms of the narrative paradigm alone.

Fisher (1987:114) acknowledges that human beings are not identical and do not share the same values, that '[w]hether through perversity, divine inspiration, or genetic programming', people make different choices and these choices 'will not be bound by ideal or "perfect" value systems – except of their own making'. The idea that values are of people's

---

[5] www.telegraph.co.uk/news/2020/08/26/will-have-generation-scarred-children-telegraph-readers-face/.

own making leaves the issue of how we come to embrace certain values rather than others rather vague. And while the narrative paradigm suggests that different values that inform the choices we make are a product of the narratives we come to believe in, Fisher does not directly explain why we come to believe in specific narratives rather than others, beyond stating that 'the production and practice of good reasons', which is informed by the narratives we subscribe to, 'is ruled by matters of history, biography, culture, and character' (Fisher 1985b:75).

The concept of narrative accrual (Bruner 1991) can shed some light on the process by which certain values come to be ratified through the accrual of a network of related narratives to which we are repeatedly exposed over time. As we have seen in the previous section, the media – including social media – constitute an important site through which particular types of narrative accrue and come to impact the values of those exposed to them over time. Other such sites include the family, circle of friends, the educational system, professional groups, the film and videogaming industry and religious institutions, among others. Narrative accrual validates certain values and invalidates others over an individual's lifetime, with networks of related narratives ultimately combining to form a tradition or (sub)culture whose members share a similar outlook on life. The (transcendental) values we acquire through this process become so ingrained that questioning them threatens our very sense of identity and ability to make sense of the world.

Alongside narrative accrual, there is also our basic human need to feel part of a community with a shared outlook on life. McClure (2009:204) thus suggests that 'many widely accepted narratives that defy both probability and fidelity' can only be understood by appeal to the concept of identification. Fisher does draw on this concept in developing his model, but as Stroud (2016) explains, he 'casts identification as an outcome when a reader encounters a narrative that is judged to be high in narrative probability and narrative fidelity'. Stroud sees this as a strength of the narrative paradigm, but McClure (2009:198) convincingly argues that it restricts 'processes of identification to the normative criteria of the rational-world', 'unnecessarily limits our understanding of the rhetoricality of narrative' (McClure 2009:191) and hence underestimates 'the irrational resources of identification, those "puzzlements and ambiguities," those "enthymemic elements," and those "partially 'unconscious' factors" that are at work in the everyday narratives by which we live' (McClure 2009:199). We follow McClure in treating identification not as an outcome of a successful test of probability and narrative fidelity, but rather as part of the definition of good reasons, acknowledging, with him (McClure 2009:202), that '[w]hat changes by reconceptualizing identification in the narrative paradigm, is what counts as "good reasons." And what counts as good reasons is identification'.

3.2.1 The Logic of Good Reasons, Narrative Accrual and Identification: Public Safety and Structural Racism

A strong cultural association between thugs, gangsters and face coverings has been gradually ratified in Anglophone and European societies through the accrual of a whole range of narratives to which we are repeatedly exposed through various sites and media. This cultural association has been evident in the context of the current pandemic, for instance when concerns are raised with respect to whether the use of face masks for medical purposes might pose a threat to public safety. A New York based lawyer, Kevin O'Brien, posed the question in a blog post titled 'Are coronavirus policies aiding criminal activity?' (O'Brien

2020). His answer points to the structural and material incoherence that exists between anti-masking laws still in force in several American states and pro-mask regulations in the context of Covid-19. While acknowledging that anti-masking laws have exacerbated social injustices, as in cases where they have been used 'to arrest masked Antifa members for the act of wearing a mask, even where they have not committed any violent acts', O'Brien also claims that these laws 'aid law enforcement in numerous ways'. He backs this claim by referring to criminological studies demonstrating that anonymity is 'commonly linked to deviant behavior' and goes on to argue:

> But the result of these Coronavirus compliant policy changes appears to be immediate, and dramatic – with the vast majority of people wearing masks, it is extremely difficult for law enforcement to identify who is inciting the violence, particularly when they are not members of the local community. I might be able to recognize my neighbor in a mask and a hood, but could I identify a stranger? Without this method of tying a specific individual to a specific act, elected officials and others seem to be more prone to speculate as to who is behind the violence and people seem more likely to commit crime.
>
> Whatever you think of current recommendations and mandates regarding masks to combat Coronavirus, it seems these decisions are making it easier for some individuals to anonymously break the law – increasing the risk for communities that public health policies are designed to protect.

Newspaper headlines linking face masks to criminal activities also contribute to the steady accrual and hence resonance of this narrative. An article in *The Telegraph* published on 21 March 2021 and entitled 'Gang members wearing coronavirus medical masks to disguise themselves' (Lowe 2020) reinforces the narrative of medical masks being used by people with criminal intentions to evade police detection. The article quotes a charity officer who works with high-risk offenders across the southeast of England arguing that face masks might be used to support anti-social behaviour: 'There could be some level of disorder in terms of anti-social behaviour. Just today in Wood Green, a young offender came up to me wearing a protective mask and offered me some marijuana'.

This link between criminal activity and masking is particularly associated with citizens who are (perceived to be) of non-Western origin – those who are classed in nationalistic narratives as 'non-indigenous'. In April 2020, the Franklin County Public Health Board in Ohio released a document addressed to 'communities of colour' about wearing face masks that they were later forced to withdraw (Franklin County Public Health 2020). The document advised black Americans to avoid using face coverings made of 'fabrics that elicit deeply held stereotypes': 'It is not recommended to wear a scarf just simply tied around the head as this can indicate unsavoury behaviour, although not intended'. The Franklin County Public Health later tweeted an apology and admitted the guidance 'came across as offensive and blaming the victims' (Figure 3.2).[6] Still, well intentioned or otherwise, such statements can impact the values of all who come across them, but particularly those to whom they are addressed and who are singled out in this narrative as a source of concern for the community and hence as positioned outside it. Importantly, they restrict the ability of such addressees to identify with the larger community and see its welfare as coherent with their own, and to view the advice given by its institutions as 'represent[ing] accurate

---

[6] https://twitter.com/fc_publichealth/status/1263187130647490561?s=21

assertions about social reality and thereby constitut[ing] good reasons for belief or action' (Fisher 1987:105).

Black citizens, in turn, have reportedly been hesitant to wear a mask in public because of the racist fears it evokes. A black physician in Boston raises the issue of how the act of making face masks mandatory in public might affect people of colour in a blog post titled

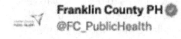

Franklin County PH ✔
@FC_PublicHealth

...

An apology from us.

Franklin County Public Health apologizes for a recent guidance document focused on mask coverings for African Americans. Some of the language used came across as offensive and blaming the victims. We have listened to the opinions that have been expressed and are using the voice of the public to inform any new guidance we put out. Everyone deserves to feel safe while wearing a face covering and not be subjected to stigma, bias or discrimination. We apologize and will continue to stay engaged in tough conversations to be better for the communities we serve.

9:17 PM · May 20, 2020 · Twitter Web App

Figure 3.2 Franklin County Public Health Board apology

'Wearing a face mask helps protect me against Covid-19, but not against racism' (Felix 2020):

> As a physician, I favor things that will help reduce the transmission of coronavirus infections. But as a Black man, I wondered how this order will affect people who look like me. I wondered if this order went into effect with any understanding of the fear and anxiety it could inflict on people of color.
>
> That might sound irrational to some. But it resonates with many Black people, who are far too familiar with having to interact with law enforcement for appearing 'suspicious' and in many instances having to fear for their life during these interactions.

Felix details how, being not only black but also 6 feet two inches tall, his 'decision-making' process had to be quite complex: '[it] went as far as limiting how often I went out after dark, knowing that some people will see a masked Black man as a threat'. Such cultural stereotypes and the racist anxieties they evoke are deeply embedded in a larger narrative of white supremacy that has accrued over many centuries, a narrative that assigns inferior status to numerous communities who are repeatedly cast as a source of threat to the nation proper. Zine (2020) thus argues that 'the concept of white privilege can be related to how COVID-19 mask-wearing is seen differently when worn on racialized bodies'. While masked black faces are associated with criminality, masked Asian faces are seen as an emblem of the crisis itself. 'Instead of representing a good citizen helping to stop the spread of a possible contagion, a protective mask transforms Asian bodies into the source of contagion'. Zine further points to the structural incoherence of the French mandate to wear masks which has not been accompanied by a lifting of the ban on women wearing a niqab, citing the French researcher Fatima Khemilat's comment on the irony of this situation:

> If you are Muslim and you hide your face for religious reasons, you are liable to a fine and a citizenship course where you will be taught what it is to be a good citizen . . . But if you are a non-Muslim citizen in the pandemic, you are encouraged and forced as a 'good citizen' to adopt 'barrier gestures' to protect the national community.

A similar irony – or structural incoherence in Fisher's terms – has pervaded the discourse of European leaders. In 2018, well before the outbreak of the pandemic, Boris Johnson stated that as a Member of Parliament he felt 'fully entitled' to see the faces of his constituents, describing women who wore the niqab as looking like letterboxes and bank robbers.[7] And yet, as noted in an article titled 'Veiled racism: how the law change on Covid-19 face coverings makes Muslim women feel', published in *The Independent* on 26 June (Begum 2020),

> [f]rom 15 June 2020, Boris Johnson – the same politician who caused a wave of anti-Muslim sentiment with his column in 2018 – has made it mandatory that all people in England wear face coverings on public transport. As well as encouraging them in other places it is hard to social distance like shops or supermarkets. The government even issued guidelines on how to make your own face covering at home.

These and similar inconsistencies in policies and statements by political leaders serve to amplify racist fears and anxieties among those who are exposed to them and undercut the

---

[7] www.bbc.co.uk/news/uk-politics-45083275.

possibility of identification with the larger community among those cast as threatening to the nation's way of life and security. Black, Asian and Muslim members of these societies who do not comply with mandatory measures such as wearing face masks in public areas, or who do so under duress and without believing that applying these measures is genuinely in their interest, are not 'irrational'. Their behaviour is informed by considerations that are narratively – if not scientifically – rational and that reflect their own lived experience, both prior to and during the pandemic. Ultimately, as Marcus (2020) argues, 'combatting racism is inextricable from public health', as indeed are so many social issues such as poverty, unemployment, trust in political and social institutions, and much else.

3.2.2 Good Reasons, Precarious Manhood and Homophobia

Identification, as McClure (2009:202) argues, constitutes good reasons for action and belief in and of itself. The examples of racism against black, Asian and Muslim people discussed above suggest that those at the receiving end of racism will find it difficult to identify with the larger community and trust its institutions. Similarly, narratives of masculinity and homophobia may serve to pressurize those socialized into them to act in ways that are consistent with the values they promote and that have been reinforced during the crisis by high-profile personalities, as we detail below. In other words, they pressurize them to behave in ways that are ratified by the group with which they identify.

Masculinity and homophobia have impacted responses to face masking during the Covid-19 crisis in various ways. Narratives that cast heterosexual men as strong, hardened, no-nonsense members of the 'real' community and gay men as effeminate, feeble and repulsive have been accruing in all societies around the world for centuries. Many men, in all cultures, are socialized to varying degrees into thinking that manhood is a highly desirable character trait and tend to associate it with physical strength and fearlessness. This 'performative masculinity', as Abad-Santos (2020) calls it, rests on 'a narrow vision of manhood that ignores other tropes like self-sacrifice and being a protector', but it has proved very powerful during the pandemic. As *The New York Times* acknowledges,[8] 'the best public health practices have collided with several of the social demands men in many cultures are pressured to follow to assert their masculinity: displaying strength instead of weakness, showing a willingness to take risks, hiding their fear, appearing to be in control'. And indeed, numerous polls have shown that many more men than women refuse to wear face masks, most notably in the USA, urging commentators like Abad-Santos (2020) to ask in disbelief:

> Fellas, is it gay[9] to not die of a virus that turns your lungs into soggy shells of their former selves, drowning you from the inside out? Is wearing a mask to avoid death part of the feminization of America? Is it too emasculating to wear a mask to protect the others around you? Does staying alive make you feel weak?

Persistent socialization into the dominant narrative of masculinity means not only that manhood is understood as 'innate', something a 'real' man is born with, but also that it is 'simultaneously precarious and in need of defending', leading those who value masculinity

---

[8] www.nytimes.com/2020/10/10/us/politics/trump-biden-masks-masculinity.html.
[9] 'Fellas, is it gay' is a series of ironic tweets that went viral in 2017, with variations such as 'Fellas, is it gay to take out the trash'. See https://knowyourmeme.com/memes/fellas-is-it-gay.

to 'overperform' their manhood and 'police its lack in others' (McBee 2019). Refusing to wear face masks and ridiculing others who do provided an opportunity for many to demonstrate their manhood during the crisis, encouraged by high-profile male personalities engaged in their own overperformance of manhood. In October 2020, for instance, *The New York Times* reported that Joe Biden posted a picture of himself on Twitter wearing a mask, in response to which 'Tomi Lahren, a conservative commentator and Fox Nation host' declared that Biden 'might as well carry a purse with that mask'.[10] Some evangelists in the USA called men who chose to wear face masks '"losers," "pansies" and "no balls"' (Harsin 2020:1065). The Brazilian President Jair Bolsonaro is reported in the leading broadsheet *Folha de São Paulo* to have 'baited presidential staff who were using protective masks, claiming such equipment was "coisa de viado" (a homophobic slur that roughly translates as "for fairies")' (Phillips 2020). The same broadsheet reported that despite the alarming spread of the virus in Brazil at the time, 'Bolsonaro insisted on greeting visitors with a handshake and shunned masks'. This brand of 'toxic white masculinity', as Harsin describes it, was 'showcased in some popular COVID-19 responses (Trump, Bolsonaro and Orban, most spectacularly)', and can be 'described as "toxic" or "fragile"' because it is 'threatened by anything associated with perceived femininity; it is further associated with physical strength, sexual conquest, a lack of any emotions signifying vulnerability (except for aggressive ones), domination, control and violence' (Harsin 2020:1063).

In an article in *Scientific American*, Willingham (2020) called masks 'condoms of the face', comparing men's resistance to wearing masks to their refusal to use condoms during the HIV pandemic. Willingham explains this resistance in terms of a 'white masculine ideology' associated with adventure, risk and violence, whose 'high priest' is Donald Trump. By refusing to wear masks, men who have been socialized to think of themselves in these terms 'expect that their masculine ideology group will accept them, respect them and not reject them'. The editor of the conservative religious journal *First Things*, R. R. Reno, defended the rejection of face masks in terms that confirm Willingham's analysis: in one out of a series of tweets (that were later erased) he insisted that '[t]he mask culture is fear driven. Masks + cowardice. It's a regime dominated by fear of infection and fear of causing of infection. Both are species of cowardice' (quoted in Kristian 2020). In a subsequent tweet, Reno challenged his audience to declare themselves fearless or cowardly. 'There are those who are terrified, and those who are not. Where do you stand?'. Like the Young Earth Creationists McClure uses to exemplify how narrative identification works, many men continue to invest in white masculine ideology because 'rejecting it has the implication of undermining the larger narrative(s) of which it is a part and rejecting the larger community to which they belong' (McClure 2009:207).

Julia Marcus, an epidemiologist at Harvard Medical School, argues in an article in *The Atlantic* that public health authorities should acknowledge and address such values rather than condemning them. 'Acknowledging what people dislike about a public-health strategy enables a connection with them rather than alienating them further', she suggests (Marcus 2020). Like Willingham (2020), she compares men's refusal to wear face masks with their reluctance to wear condoms during the HIV pandemic. Just as companies began to make condoms that not only protect people but also address their need for pleasure and intimacy, she argues, governments should now 'support businesses in developing masks that are not only effective, but ... that make them feel

---

[10] www.nytimes.com/2020/10/10/us/politics/trump-biden-masks-masculinity.html.

stylish, cool, and – yes – even manly' (Marcus 2020). This is sound advice, as far as it goes, and following it could make wearing masks more palatable for some of those who regard them as 'unmanly', though it arguably also runs the risk of giving more credence and legitimacy to toxic masculinity. More importantly, unlike condoms, masks are worn in public and hence exacerbate the need for 'precarious manhood' to be asserted. The implications of wearing them or otherwise are further complicated by their association with specific political positions, leading a public health professor at Morgan State University in the USA to comment that '[w]e're seeing politics and science literally clashing'. The BBC news report that quotes him agrees (McKelvey 2020):

> The wearing of masks has become a catalyst for political conflict, an arena where scientific evidence is often viewed through a partisan lens. Most Democrats support the wearing of masks, according to a poll conducted by researchers at the Pew Research Center.
>   Most Republicans do not.

Writing some two months later (in August of the same year), Abad-Santos (2020) reports that sports companies like Nike and Under Armor are already 'making masks that superheroes might don', including some that are curved like shark fins and one, by GQ, that makes its wearer look like he's 'in Mortal Kombat'. Abad-Santos points to a further complication that undermines the value of attempts to appeal to masculine imagery in order to encourage more men to wear masks. 'For men concerned with masculinity, the appeal here is that these masks not only look cool but allow you to do masculine things like run faster, lift heavier, and be stronger'. This means that manufacturers use porous material 'which is designed to be breathable and in fact breaks up larger particles, allowing them to hang around in the air longer', and making people wear these masks is possibly worse than them not wearing masks at all (according to Abad-Santos). Any advice on how to address resistance to face masks must therefore consider a wide range of factors that have arguably made the Covid-19 crisis more challenging to public health policy makers than most pandemics humanity has faced in the past.

3.3 Beyond Precariousness: Personal Freedom vs Social Responsibility

Perhaps the most fundamental value commitment underpinning the debates about face coverings is the notion of individual freedom. Controversies around different understandings of this transcendental value, as well as how it relates to social responsibility, have dominated much of the current debate, implicitly or explicitly. Anti-mask protests have occurred in many countries in response to mask mandates, some claiming that such mandates 'sacrifice individual liberty to a collectivist notion of a "greater good"' (Blunt 2020). The conception of 'freedom as non-interference' that inspires these protests has also elicited support from prominent figures on the political right in the UK and America: Peter Hitchens of the *Daily Mail*, for instance, referred to face coverings as 'muzzles' (Hitchins 2020) while Michael Savage, a prominent radio talk host, called masks 'a sign of submission' (Walker 2020).

   Similar 'us' vs 'them' dichotomies have been implicitly evoked to argue that the use of face masks might be acceptable for certain populations but is at odds with the values of freedom underpinning Anglophone and European societies. Having denounced face masks as 'muzzles', Peter Hitchins went on to declare that their mandatory use marked

> the final closing down of centuries of human liberty and the transformation of one of the freest countries on Earth [the UK] into a regimented, conformist society, under perpetual surveillance, in which a subservient people scurries about beneath the stern gaze of authority.

In a blog post on the Architects for Social Housing website, entitled 'The science and law of refusing to wear masks: texts and arguments in support of civil disobedience', Elmer (2020) considers the general use of face masks in Asian countries against the backdrop of the 'arsenal of surveillance tools' available to the governments of China, Hong Kong, South Korea and Taiwan to track and monitor their populations. As part of this arsenal, he lists the mass surveillance of mobile phone, rail, credit card and flight data, including the use of 'facial recognition algorithms to identify commuters who aren't wearing a mask or who aren't wearing one properly', among many other such intrusive practices. These technologies of surveillance, he argues, are now being advocated for use in the West and must be confronted through civil disobedience if necessary. Elmer supports his claim by quoting an article published in the influential *Foreign Affairs* by Nicholas Wright, a UK medical doctor and neuroscientist, in which he (Wright) insists that 'Western democracies must rise to meet the need for "democratic surveillance" to protect their own populations', that 'they must be unafraid in trying to sharpen their powers of surveillance for public health purposes', and that 'there is nothing oxymoronic about the idea of "democratic surveillance"' (N. Wright 2020). Elmer then rebuts Wright's argument by recalling the words of Giorgio Agamben, the well-known Italian philosopher who criticized the Italian government's use of the coronavirus as a warrant for implementing a permanent state of emergency (Agamben 2021:48):

> A norm which affirms that we must renounce the good to save the good is as false and contradictory as that which, in order to protect freedom, imposes the renunciation of freedom.

Some have linked this debate about face masks and protecting vs renouncing freedom to the distinction between negative and positive liberty, freedom *from* vs freedom *to*. This distinction, which underpins two opposing sets of transcendental values – both narratively rational and both providing good reasons for their adherents – goes back to Kant, who distinguished between freedom understood in negative terms as an absence of constraints, and freedom understood in positive terms as the possibility of auto-commencement (self-beginning, or *Selbstanfang*), in the sense of acting and taking control of one's life. As the *Stanford Encyclopedia of Philosophy* explains, 'While negative liberty is usually attributed to individual agents, positive liberty is sometimes attributed to collectivities, or to individuals considered primarily as members of given collectivities'.[11] An appeal to positive liberty would sanction state intervention where required, whereas an appeal to negative liberty would favour placing strong restrictions on state intervention. In political philosophy, the classical liberal tradition, represented by philosophers such as Spencer and Mill, is seen as defending a negative concept of political freedom, while theorists critical of this tradition,

---

[11] https://plato.stanford.edu/entries/liberty-positive-negative/.

such as Rousseau and Marx, are associated with a positive concept of political freedom. Munroe (2020) implicitly sides with the latter view when in a commentary in *The Herald* he draws on this distinction to demonstrate how the debate about face masks brings the two understandings of freedom into conflict:

> Requiring individuals to wear a face mask under penalty of fines does deprive them of a negative liberty, but it strengthens a greater liberty which can only be protected through coordinated public action, it creates conditions by which we can all safely access social services and businesses.

For Agamben, however, the freedom renounced through wearing face coverings goes beyond the negative definition of absence of constraints. Agamben sees the mandate of covering the face as a threat to the very condition of politics and the positive freedom of humans as political beings. While animals do not acknowledge their exposure or consider it a problem, as 'they simply dwell in it without caring about it', human beings 'want to recognise themselves and to be recognised, they want to appropriate their own image, seeking in it their own truth' (Agamben 2020). The face, according to Agamben, is 'the place of politics', it is what reveals true investment in an argument and translates pieces of information into statements: 'If individuals only had to communicate information on this or that thing, there would never be proper politics, but only an exchange of messages' (Agamben 2021:87). Based on this notion of politics, he concludes that 'a country that decides to give up its own face, to cover the faces of its citizens with masks everywhere is, then, a country that has erased all political dimensions from itself' (Agamben 2021:87).

Ultimately, as Christos Lynteris – a medical anthropologist at the University of St Andrews in Scotland – notes, the reasons for failing or openly refusing to wear a mask are many and complex (Goodman 2020). In addition to the values and logics already discussed in this chapter, there are young people who are convinced that Covid-19 is an old people's disease and cannot or is highly unlikely to affect them, leading them to treat it as a common cold or the flu; there are others for whom 'refusal to wear a mask has become a visual symbol of being a free-thinker and nonconformist' (Lynteris, in Goodman 2020); and there are others still who think masks are for Asians, not 'us', and are 'a tool of communist control' (Lynteris, in Goodman 2020). Whatever the beliefs that these individuals and communities entertain about wearing face masks, they are as rational to them as any piece of evidence-based scientific advice. They are strongly held because they are informed by narratives and values that have been acquired and reinforced through ongoing processes of socialization, by the need to identify with a particular community and by their own lived experience. The latter directly impacts the extent to which narratives about the benefits of wearing a mask and other health-related information may or may not resonate with particular publics such as the black community.

Whose Lives? What Values? Herd Immunity, Lockdowns and Social/ Physical Distancing

As in the case of face masking, disagreements about mass public health measures such as lockdowns and physical distancing have dominated the discussion around Covid-19. Policy-oriented discourses such as recommendations and media briefings have argued for more or less severe measures, ranging from national curfews to mandated social distancing, or mitigation strategies built on the premise of quickly reaching herd immunity. All these different measures have been extensively debated in the media and other public forums and continuously monitored by international organizations such as the World Health Organization, the US Centers for Disease Control and Prevention and European Centre for Disease Prevention and Control. Policy arguments have also been revised or refocused in tandem with a growing body of research and natural experiments as countries began to introduce either mandatory or voluntary policies. This chapter examines various arguments deployed in this debate and the complex dialogue between political, scientific and popular values and discourses.

It is fair to say at the outset that, once again, at least some of the resistance to such measures can be explained by the structural and material incoherence of public policy in many areas of the world. As Devi Sridhar, Chair of Global Public Health at the University of Edinburgh, explains (Sridhar 2020), in the case of the UK the late imposition of a full lockdown followed by cycles of short lockdowns, which were not accompanied by an effective test and trace strategy, with people actively encouraged to go abroad on holidays in between these short lockdowns, left many exhausted and confused. Hence, she concludes:

> It's no surprise that those offering easy, compelling solutions – 'You can have your life back by Christmas'; 'It's either the economy or health'; 'This virus is practically harmless to those under 55'; have found a willing audience in a frustrated and fatigued society.

Hickman (2020), Professor of Public Law at University College London, has similarly argued that public policies have obscured the distinction between advice and information about legal prohibitions, which has led to a form of material incoherence that he calls 'normative ambiguity':

> This phenomenon meant that the scope of individual liberty was unclear and at times misrepresented. Whilst the coronavirus guidance was drafted to fulfil well-intentioned public health objectives, by implying, even unintentionally, that criminal law restrictions were different or more extensive than they in fact were and by failing accurately to delineate the boundary between law and advice, the coronavirus guidance failed to respect individual autonomy in a fundamental way.

Furthermore, the arguments supporting the need for and the measures adopted in the implementation of restrictions have been interpreted and applied very differently in various areas of the world, giving some the impression that the measures imposed on different populations are arbitrary and indeed not to be trusted. Early in the pandemic, China introduced a full-blown lockdown in several provinces and imposed very strong measures of control, including barricading of villages, hiring of community guardians, financial rewards for reporting those who broke lockdown regulations and phone apps to track the movement of citizens (Feng and Chen 2020). Several European countries, including Spain and France, also introduced formal curfews forbidding citizens to leave their homes. In Spain, even children under 14 were not allowed to leave their home for a period of six weeks (Hedgecoe 2020), placing immense pressure on them as well as their parents. The level of stress caused by extended confinement varied considerably, depending on the nature of the space in which families experienced the lockdown. Those higher up the social and economic scale, who had more room to work and live, naturally experienced lockdowns and curfews differently from those whose living space was more restricted. As one contributor to a Twitter exchange about the wisdom of lockdowns put it, 'Lockdown is a luxury of the middle classes. . . . Middle classes work from their gardens'.

At the other extreme, the Norwegian government's attempt to introduce an emergency bill allowing the imposition of a limited curfew for a few hours a day, and only in extreme cases, was defeated even before reaching Parliament due to massive public resistance. Similarly, Sweden built its strategy on responsibility and trust rather than enforced restrictions and introduced few behavioural restrictions compared to most other countries (Orange 2020). The UK's approach to lockdown perhaps constitutes the starkest example of structural incoherence and led to widespread confusion and loss of trust. It started in March 2020 with the three-point slogan 'Stay home, protect the NHS, save lives', a clear message that was well received, in part because the National Health Service (NHS) is a widely trusted and much loved institution with which a majority of British people readily identify. In May 2020, however, this slogan was replaced with 'Stay alert, control the virus, save lives', leading to much confusion. Not only was the reference to the much loved NHS lost, but the 'stay alert' message – which replaced an action with a subjective cognitive state – was too vague. Even government ministers were unable to articulate what 'stay alert' meant in practice. Finally, the government went back to the initial slogan of 'Stay home, protect the NHS, save lives' with the third national lockdown in England in January 2021. By then, the argument supporting the need for lockdowns had lost much ground.

Some of the national differences in the way the pandemic was handled might of course reflect differences in the severity of the outbreaks across regions and nations. Importantly, however, they also reflect differences in values and priorities. Lack of attention to differences in the cultural norms and values that underpin the various measures adopted to control the pandemic may be partly responsible for the increased confusion and resistance on the part of sections of the public in various localities. At the level of policy making, the rationale for adopting any measure has to be woven within a broader narrative of the pandemic and its implications for various sections of a given community: child/adult, young/elderly, healthy/vulnerable, wealthy/poor, working/retired and so on. And given that narratives are ultimately 'symbolic interpretations of aspects of the world occurring in time and shaped by history, culture, and character' (Fisher 1987:xiii), degrees of compliance with or rejection of imposed restrictions, especially those that involve major disruption to people's daily lives, will naturally vary among locales and communities, as some of the examples we discuss in this chapter demonstrate.

4.1 Structural/Material (In)coherence *or* Science vs Values in the Great Barrington and John Snow Declarations

Structural and material incoherence in the scientific discourse about Covid-19 may be ascribed to a lack of acknowledgement of the values underpinning the adversary position rather than inconsistencies in the findings. The debate that followed the Great Barrington Declaration[1] warning against the 'damaging physical and mental health impacts of the prevailing Covid-19 policies' is a case in point. The Declaration was written by Dr Jay Bhattacharya, Dr Sunetra Gupta and Dr Martin Kulldorff and released to the public on 5 October 2020. It was originally signed by some 30+ members of the medical community but went on to attract the signatures of over 42,000 medical practitioners, over 14,000 medical and public health scientists and over 787,000 concerned citizens.[2] It recommended an approach that its original signatories dubbed 'Focused Protection' and defined as follows:

> The most compassionate approach that balances the risks and benefits of reaching herd immunity, is to allow those who are at minimal risk of death to live their lives normally to build up immunity to the virus through natural infection, while better protecting those who are at highest risk. We call this Focused Protection.[3]

Writing in *The Guardian* soon after, on 10 October, Sridhar (2020) accepts that the solution to the crisis 'cannot just be locking down continually' but points to several instances of material incoherence in the Declaration, without specifically engaging with the values that inform it:

> ... how do you distinguish the vulnerable from the healthy? This isn't just about age – Covid is proven to have worse outcomes in people who are overweight, of particular ethnicities, or have preexisting conditions they may not even be aware of.

The Declaration was soon countered by another manifesto, the John Snow Memorandum, first published in *The Lancet* on 15 October 2020 (Alwan et al. 2020) and to date boasting more than 6,900 carefully vetted signatures by scientists, researchers and healthcare professionals.[4] It argued that '[a]ny pandemic management strategy relying upon immunity from natural infections for COVID-19 is flawed'; that '[u]ncontrolled transmission in younger people risks significant morbidity and mortality across the whole population'; and that this additional human cost 'would impact the workforce as a whole and overwhelm the ability of healthcare systems to provide acute and routine care'. Its authors further dismissed the herd immunity approach as 'a dangerous fallacy unsupported by scientific evidence'. By framing the issue as a question of evidence for or against herd immunity, the debate quickly reached a dead end. Although the theory of herd immunity is embraced by the authors of the Barrington Declaration, evidence claims and arguments in its favour are almost absent from the text. The Declaration tells a different story. Driven by

---

[1] The Declaration was written and signed at the American Institute for Economic Research, Great Barrington, Massachusetts – from which location it acquired its title.
[2] https://gbdeclaration.org/view-signatures/.   [3] https://gbdeclaration.org.
[4] https://www.johnsnowmemo.com/.

a desire to 'protect people', the group wished to counter 'grave injustice' and the 'devastating effects on short and long-term public health'. The consequences of 'current lockdown policies', they argued, include

> lower childhood vaccination rates, worsening cardiovascular disease outcomes, fewer cancer screenings and deteriorating mental health – leading to greater excess mortality in years to come, with the working class and younger members of society carrying the heaviest burden.

As Cayley (2020) notes, 'whether these harms outweigh the benefits of flattening the curve is a moral question, not a scientific one'. While dismissing the validity of its scientific claims, Greenhalgh et al.'s (2020) critique of the Declaration therefore ultimately focuses on issues such as the inhumanity of shutting away the most vulnerable. It also asks questions such as 'who funded this piece of political theatre', thus casting doubt on the integrity and char-acterological coherence of those who issued the statement. Addressing the issue as an expert in political economy, Murphy (2020) uses stark images to highlight the inhumanity of what is proposed by the Declaration. What it suggests is best described as a 'cull' of the popula-tion, he states; its content has everything to do with 'far-right economics' and little to do with epidemiology or science. His article begins by reminding its readers that 'The Nazi's first victims were the disabled, which they saw as an economic drag on society', and ends by evoking a saying that has had considerable resonance in Anglophone and European soci-eties since the Second World War:

> Remember, first they came for those they deemed to be the elderly ... You can fill in the blanks.

By failing to engage with the values to which the Great Barrington Declaration appeals and focusing instead on the scientific evidence for herd immunity, the John Snow Memorandum fails to argue on the terms of rationality evoked by and relevant to the narrative elaborated by the authors of the Declaration. Furthermore, by not acknowledging the values that underpin that narrative, the authors of the Memorandum fail to address what Fisher refers to as the question of consistency, that is, 'whether the values are confirmed or validated in one's personal experience, in the lives or statements of others whom one admires and respects, and in a conception of the best audience that one can conceive' (Fisher 1987:109). In this respect, Tang (2020) does more justice to the values of the story by acknowledging them as valid, comparing the proposed approach to that already adopted to protect vulnerable sections of the population (mainly the elderly) against influenza, while pointing out the structural incoherence in the proposed 'Focused Protection' approach in the case of Covid-19, where no vaccine was yet available at the time:

> So I appreciate and understand the concerns and the sentiment behind this declaration, and of course other diseases are important and need attention, but without these anti-COVID-19 'tools' [i.e. vaccines], I cannot see how they will achieve this 'Focused Protection' for these vulnerable groups in any practical, reliable or safe way.

In asserting the need to engage with the Declaration on its own terms of rationality and address the values that underpin its narrative of the route out of the pandemic, we do not seek to support its arguments or imply that they are informed by scientific evidence. We merely wish to stress that arguments against lockdowns and other measures for which scientific evidence may be lacking can be driven by a commitment to positive values (such as concern about growing social problems and inequities among children and young people). Engaging with such arguments on their own terms rather than by recourse to lack or otherwise of scientific evidence can be crucial in creating a productive dialogue with people who hold these values.

An impression of structural and material incoherence can also result from the oversimplification or deliberate undermining of the values that underpin medical expert opinion. In September 2020, two open letters were sent to the UK's four chief medical officers expressing conflicting views among medical experts about how the government should handle the then emerging second wave of Covid-19. Sunetra Gupta, a professor of theoretical epidemiology at Oxford University, Carl Heneghan, director of the Centre for Evidence Based Medicine at Oxford, Karol Sikora, a consultant oncologist at the University of Buckingham, and 30 others called on the government to adopt a more targeted approach by shielding the most vulnerable groups in society rather than imposing local or national lockdown measures.[5] Trish Greenhalgh, a professor of primary care at the University of Oxford, published an opposing letter – endorsed by 22 colleagues – which supported the effort to suppress the virus across the entire population. This letter argued that it would be impractical to cut off a cohort of vulnerable people from the rest in an open society, stated that this is especially the case 'for disadvantaged groups (e.g. those living in cramped housing and multi-generational households)', and pointed out that '[m]any grandparents are looking after children sent home from school while parents are at work'.[6]

Interestingly, both letters – which mainly express differences in values regarding how to define and shield the most vulnerable – were met with criticism regarding lack of evidence, particularly quantitative data to support their claims, as can be seen in the following Twitter comments on the letter by Greenhalgh and colleagues:[7]

Freeman London:
I am afraid that there is little science in this response. What does this even mean? 'a) While covid-19 has different incidence and outcome in different groups, deaths have occurred in all age, gender and racial/ethnic groups and in people with no pre-existing medical conditions. Long Covid (symptoms extending for weeks or months after covid-19) is a debilitating disease affecting tens of thousands of people in UK, and can occur in previously young and healthy individuals' – Of course all cohorts are impacted but what about the numbers!? All decisions should be risk/reward based referencing scientific/analytical data. We are destroying our country from an economic, health and social perspective. Our children will pay the price for decades to come. You must see the big picture here and stop making statements like the above that have no quantitative, scientific basis.

Lesley Atkins
Well said. There has been no intelligent or systemic calibration of the impact of this virus. No thought given to the destruction of people's lives and health and well being; instead we have been subjected to a daily dose of propaganda masquerading as science.

The demand for 'science' and quantitative data to support the claim that 'deaths have occurred in all age, gender and racial/ethnic groups' arguably misses the point – namely,

---

[5] https://twitter.com/ProfKarolSikora/status/1307972101463212032.
[6] https://blogs.bmj.com/bmj/2020/09/21/covid-19-an-open-letter-to-the-uks-chief-medical-officers/.
[7] See Comments section at: blogs.bmj.com/bmj/2020/09/21/covid-19-an-open-letter-to-the-uks-chief-medical-officers/.

that vulnerable groups are not easily defined and shielded and that everyone therefore needs to be protected, whether through lockdowns or other measures. Knowledge about the exact size of the various groups affected by the virus would not add to or weaken the core argument simply because the argument is not about facts and statistics but about values. Just as the author of the Twitter post (Freeman London) does not see the need to back his claim that we are 'destroying our country from an economic, health and social perspective' by numbers because the assertion is a value statement, Greenhalgh et al.'s argument does not hinge on scientific evidence. What Greenhalgh and colleagues are ultimately suggesting is not that more or fewer lives would be lost if the argument for herd immunity wins, or that the economy is not adversely affected by lockdowns, but rather (implicitly) that *all* lives must be valued and protected, irrespective of the numbers involved and the impact of lockdowns and other restrictions on the economy. This is fundamentally a moral argument about the value of human life and recalls the experience of Dr Clarke, the palliative care doctor whose visceral account of observing the 89-year-old Winston die of Covid-19 we discussed in Chapter 2:

> You could argue – indeed, some commentators have essentially done so – that there was little point to a man like Winston. He was 89 years old, after all, and probably hadn't been economically productive for three decades. He was lucky, frankly, to have had an innings like that. Of course the young must come first. . . .
> But to those of us up close with this dreadful disease – who see, as we do, the way it suffocates the life from you – such judgments are grotesque. . . .
> Winston, though vulnerable, was loved and cherished. His death was not inevitable, his time hadn't come. He was no more disposable than any of us.

It is important to acknowledge, however, that different people can appeal to the same or similar values to support opposite points of view. Cayley (2020), for instance, argues that in framing the issue as one of not overwhelming the health system to such an extent that doctors are forced to make a decision about who lives and who dies on hospital wards, we merely mask the fact that we are quietly making similar decisions outside the hospital setting without acknowledging them:

> If someone loses a business, in which they have invested everything, and then their life falls apart, have they not been sacrificed or triaged, just as surely as the old person who we feared might not get a ventilator? Moral decisions are difficult, but they should at least be faced as moral decisions.

Giorgio Agamben, who has been a vocal critic of Covid-19 restrictions – not only lockdowns and various restrictions on mobility but also measures such as the mandatory use of face masks – also appeals to our sense of shared humanity when he argues (Agamben 2021:60):

> . . . the Church has radically disavowed its most essential principles [in the context of Covid-19]. Led by a Pope named Francis, it is forgetting that St Francis embraced the lepers. It is forgetting that one of the works of mercy is visiting the sick. It is forgetting the martyrs' teaching that we must be willing to sacrifice life rather than faith, and that renouncing one's neighbour means renouncing faith.

Interestingly, too, the argument against herd immunity is often informed by a belief in the value of autonomy and personal freedom rather than the value of all or some human lives *per se*. Many people instinctively reject the idea of 'following the herd' uncritically and prefer to think of themselves as free and independent human beings. As Larson (2020: 23) points out, the very term herd immunity 'provokes perceptions of people being herded like sheep and assuming an unquestioning herd mentality, lacking autonomy, and just doing what the "system" dictates'.

To return to the letters by Gupta et al. and Greenhalgh and colleagues, some responses to the latter used the interdependence between health and the economy to point to instances of structural/material (in)coherence, as in the following tweet, which starts with the incoherence of sacrificing the very economy on which the NHS depends for survival and then goes on to question values such as the acceptance or otherwise of a certain threshold for overall Covid-related deaths and the disregard for civil liberties:[8]

Dental Law & Ethics
Question 1) How do you 'protect the NHS' by bankrupting the country, the tax base of which is primarily used to fund the NHS? Question 2) How do the supporters of the nationwide lockdowns feel we should address the disastrous international consequences of said lockdowns. For example, the UN have stated nearly 250 million people face starvation as a direct result. Question 3) How many deaths directly attributable to the lockdown are acceptable? Spike in suicides (e.g. 500 directly related to the lockdown in Thailand in a country with less than 30 COVID deaths), 350 K people not getting the cancer care they need and the 3 million missed screenings which will see a spike in cancer deaths due to missed early treatments and diagnosis. Question 4) Why was Prof Petersons model (which has been widely criticised by anyone who got to examine the source code) so readily accepted whilst Sunetra Gupta's Oxford model was ignored? Question 5) Are those who support the lockdown regime willing to accept the loss of the civil liberties of their children going forward?

Paradoxically, an explicit aim of both letters (Gupta et al.'s and Greenhalgh's) was to argue against a polarized view. The letter by Gupta et al. argues that the debate is stuck in an 'unhelpfully polarised' deadlock between those who claim that Covid is 'extremely deadly to all' and those who believe that it 'poses no risk at all'. Greenhalgh et al. also explicitly argue against polarization:

'Facts' will be differently valued and differently interpreted by different experts and different interest groups. A research finding that is declared 'best evidence' or 'robust evidence' by one expert will be considered marginal or flawed by another expert. It is more important than ever to consider multiple perspectives on the issues and encourage interdisciplinary debate and peer review.

Unfortunately, in the heated debate that followed the publication of the two letters these values of conciliation, the need to embrace uncertainties and the importance of interdisciplinary debate – all of which are explicitly promoted by the authors of both letters – were rarely acknowledged or discussed.

A final limitation on the potential resonance of either side of the debate initiated by the two letters for large sections of the global community is, as one comment put it, that it is all

---

[8] Again, see Comments section at:https://blogs.bmj.com/bmj/2020/09/21/covid-19-an-open-letter-to-the-uks-chief-medical-officers/#comment-5080833679.

about the UK, with no consideration given to the very different environments in which the pandemic has had disastrous consequences for various sectors of society:[9]

M Lyndon
... This open letter is about the UK. In countries where people literally face starvation, lockdowns probably aren't effective. The only bright side to a very dismal picture is that such countries typically have younger populations and lower rates of diabetes and obesity.

Writing on the London School of Economics blog early in the outbreak, on 27 March, Broadbent and Smart (2020) were already aware of differences in the way restrictions on mobility would be experienced in various parts of the world. They argued that a one-size fits all approach cannot work, and focusing especially on Africa and the potential for widespread starvation they pointed out:

The crunch question is this: what is the case fatality rate of social distancing in Africa? We have no idea; but that is the figure that should be considered when implementing social distancing measures. The scientific community, including both epidemiologists and economists working together, should be putting as much effort into estimating that case fatality rate as into estimating it for COVID-19.

In addition to fatalities resulting from potential starvation, Broadbent and Smart (2020) further highlight the impracticalities of social distancing in some parts of a country such as South Africa, where there is a very high level of interdependency among households:

In a South African township, living conditions are extremely crowded. Socialising is unavoidable. You might as well tell people to emigrate to Mars. In the bubonic plague, the aristocracy left London for the countryside; the poor of London could not isolate themselves, and so they died. This may be our situation.

The living conditions they describe are not restricted to South African townships but are typical of many parts of the world, as well as within certain communities in Europe and the USA. Alser et al. (2020) make a similar argument in relation to the particularly dire situation in Gaza, which has already suffered a prolonged blockade since 2007:

Unlike the 'one size fits all' approach, measures that have proven successful in other countries might not be effective in densely populated and disadvantaged environments such as Gaza. Avoiding social gatherings or observing the two-metre distancing measure could well be viewed as foreign concepts and its effectiveness will be limited among Palestinian extended families living in overcrowded refugee camps.

Other interdependencies go beyond individual households and extended families; these interdependencies connect the city with the informal settlements that often provide it with vital services. Talking about the challenges involved in implementing Covid-related restrictions in Sierra Leone slums, Wilkinson (2020) points out that

Informal settlements and their residents are part and parcel of the city system, often subsidising and contributing to life elsewhere in the city. This makes control efforts built

---

[9] Once again, see Comments section at: https://blogs.bmj.com/bmj/2020/09/21/covid-19-an-open-letter-to-the-uks-chief-medical-officers/.

on containment and reductions in movement difficult to implement, especially if they impinge on people's already threadbare livelihoods.

Narratives revolving around the wisdom or otherwise of lockdowns and other restrictions that take no account of the specific social, political and cultural realities of a given population clearly will not resonate for members of that population and will not be seen as coherent from their perspective. However scientifically valid and rational they are, the lived experience of each community will ultimately determine its response to such measures and its ability to abide by them. In Fisher's terms, narratives that are at odds with our immediate experience of the world will be seen as lacking in both probability and fidelity. Inhabitants of a South African township or a Gaza refugee camp will see the contradictions inherent in a narrative that asserts the need to abide by social distancing given the physical reality in which they live, and will judge it as lacking in material coherence. The narrative will also not fare better from the perspective of the logic of good reasons, and especially the third criterion of *consequence*, as we defined it in Chapter 2 (Baker 2006:152):

> This criterion focuses on the real world consequences of accepting the values elaborated in the narrative. Here, we ask '[w]hat would be the effects of adhering to the values – for one's concept of oneself, for one's behavior, for one's relationships with others and society, and to the process of rhetorical transaction?'.

Similar considerations will be at play in assessing narratives that attempt to negotiate the tension between health and the economy from a variety of other perspectives.

4.2 Health, the Economy and the State: Resonance and Lived Experience

The tension between health and economic priorities has featured in many debates and venues beyond the sources discussed above, and beyond the medical establishment. Bolsover's (2020) analysis of pro- and anti-restriction discourse on social media in the USA from the early phase of the pandemic cites angry tweets that are concerned about the impact of lockdowns and other restrictions on small businesses:

> Had to stop at the local Walmart today. It was PACKED. Just goes to show you how unethical this lockdown is. I can go to a packed Walmart to buy art supplies but I can't go to the tiny local art store to buy art supplies. The disproportionate hit to small businesses is criminal.

Others point out that at the same time as these restrictions are hitting small businesses hard, they are benefitting big companies hugely, especially online companies like Amazon, in the process bringing up the issue of control over the media and the power of big business to shape policy:

> Lockdown increases Bezos wealth by tens of billions, who would have guessed that Amazon would benefit from hundreds of millions of other businesses closing down worldwide – many never to reopen? The Bezos-owned Washington Post says 'Lockdowns must continue'.

Even those who argue for lockdowns share the concern with the growing wealth and influence of big companies:

> It's wild to me that people think lockdowns are corporate/government conspiracies. The conspiracy you should be worried about is one where everyone is told that it's safe to

resume daily life as usual, when it's not, because fucking Walmart is worried about their bottom line.

In addition to the impact of restrictions on small as opposed to big businesses, some of the debate has also revolved around the distinction between essential and non-essential businesses, where areas of structural and material incoherence could be identified and questioned. Henry (2021) contests the distinction, arguing that 'small businesses are deemed non-essential, yet they provide the same products that essential, big-box stores sell on their shelves', and concludes that '[a]ll businesses should remain essential with mandatory social distance measures, capacity limits, and necessary safety protocols, so permanent closures and lay-offs are no longer a trend'. Some of the tweets cited in Bolsover (2020) question the distinction between essential and non-essential services and institutions beyond the sphere of (corporate) business, in ways that reveal deep-seated mistrust of the official institutions in the USA:

> Does anyone else find it ironic that we are all on lockdown, and businesses are closed, just to try and save lives, yet abortion clinics are still open? #openohionow

The debate about the relative importance of health vs the economy has thus tended to spill out into other areas of political, religious and social life where tensions of various kinds have been fermenting for many years. These tensions may be behind a lack of trust in the same institutions now elaborating particular narratives that promote measures such as lockdowns. And since any narrative is ultimately a story of values, as Fisher asserts, the third criterion that informs the logic of good reasons, namely *consistency*, is not met from the perspective of those members of society who mistrust these institutions. For the criterion of consistency – as we have already pointed out – requires a positive answer to the question: 'Are the values [that explicitly or implicitly inform the narrative] confirmed or validated in one's personal experience, in the lives or statements of *others whom one admires and respects*' (Fisher 1987:109; emphasis added) and, we might add, *whom one trusts*. Lack of trust in the institutions that promote and impose restrictive measures such as lockdowns also means that these institutions lack characterological coherence, in Fisher's terms. The narratives they promote are therefore not accepted as reliable or genuinely intended to safeguard the interests of the population.

Some of the protests against lockdowns and other restrictions focused specifically on their impact on the livelihoods of ordinary people rather than the economy as such. This represented a major concern and a good reason (in Fisher's terms) for questioning the wisdom and necessity of lockdowns from the perspective of the lived experience of a large section of all populations. Even in wealthy countries like the UK, '[t]he biggest victims of lockdowns and curfews have been blue-collar workers, the self-employed and those whose livelihoods depend on servicing the better-heeled in the metropolises of early 21st-century capitalism' (Coman 2020). But as we have already seen to some extent in the previous section and as Carothers and Press (2020) point out, the livelihood argument against lockdowns was particularly strong in developing countries, 'which have larger informal sectors where economic margins are thinner and remote work is often impossible'. In April 2020, Aljazeera reported that thousands of street vendors in Malawi marched with banners such as 'Lockdown more poisonous than corona' and 'We'd rather die of corona than of hunger'.[10] In Kampala, the capital of

---

[10] www.aljazeera.com/economy/2020/04/16/informal-vendors-rally-against-coronavirus-lockdown-in-malawi/.

Uganda, street vendors likewise continued to scurry to the windows of vehicles in traffic lights and jams, without masks. For them, isolating at home meant starving to death: 'The street is their workplace, livelihood and home' (Anguyo and Storer 2020). In South Africa, those working in particularly vulnerable sectors such as hospitality and retail 'protested against limitations on in-person operations' (Carothers and Press 2020). Protests that focused on the impact of restrictions on livelihoods often turned violent: 'In Lagos, Nigeria, a police spokesman said that workers in the Lekki Free Trade Zone had assaulted police, injuring several officers, after being told they could not work due to public health measures' (Carothers and Press 2020). In Malawi – 'one of the poorest countries on the continent where more than half of the population live below the poverty threshold' – civil rights organizations applied for a court order to stop the government implementing the lockdown, citing 'the government's failure to announce any measures to cushion the poor'.[11] In countries with a very high level of poverty, the issue of individual livelihoods therefore featured very prominently and invited strong responses (Figure 4.1). Arguments about the impact of restrictions on the economy as a whole, or on small vs big businesses and essential vs non-essential services, were relatively

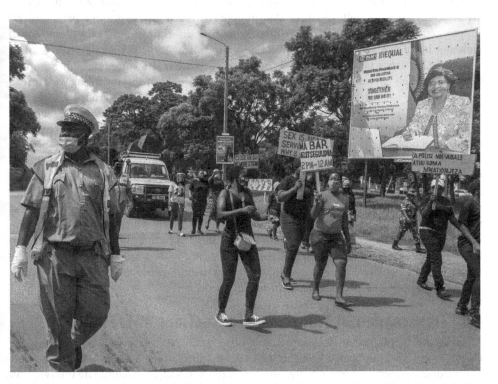

Figure 4.1 Malawi sex workers protest restrictions on opening times of bars during Covid-19 crisis, 28 January 2021. AMOS GUMULIRA / Contributor / Getty Images.

[11] www.aljazeera.com/economy/2020/04/16/informal-vendors-rally-against-coronavirus-lockdown-in-malawi/.

less prominent, reflecting the importance of visceral, lived experience – rather than abstract arguments about health vs the economy – on people's immediate assessment of the validity of Covid-related narratives.

The lived experience of populations who had reason to mistrust the state and official institutions also played a major role in shaping their responses to Covid-related restrictions. Carothers and Press (2020) point out that a recurrent theme in anti-lockdown protests concerned a perceived harshness and inconsistency in the way lockdowns were enforced and a misuse of the new rules by different regimes 'for repressive ends'. The Freedom House 2020 report, 'Democracy under lockdown' (Repucci and Slipowitz 2020), acknowledges that the crisis of democratic governance around the world predated the pandemic, but points out that many governments 'are also using the pandemic as a justification to grant themselves special powers beyond what is reasonably necessary to protect public health'. In Egypt, the military regime 'used COVID-19 as an opportunity to further repress political activists, rights defenders, lawyers, journalists, and doctors, arresting dozens, denying them basic assistance in places of detention, and placing several on terrorist lists' (Repucci and Slipowitz 2020). Liberia, likewise, witnessed a 'brutal and corrupt enforcement of curfew orders by security forces', and in Zimbabwe, the pandemic gave the authorities licence 'to arrest, abduct, rape, assault, and intimidate human rights activists, opposition party leaders/ supporters, civil society leaders, journalists, and other dissenting voices on "allegations of violating lockdown conditions"' (Repucci and Slipowitz 2020). In Uganda, '[t]he violent arrest of 23 citizens taking refuge in a shelter serving the LGBT community in Kampala, targeted for their alleged "public gathering"', similarly raised concern regarding widespread discrimination against lesbian, gay, bisexual and transgender (LGBT) groups (Storer and Dawson 2020). Elsewhere, lockdown measures were selectively enforced on some segments of the population rather than others. For example, in Bulgaria 'Romany neighborhoods were placed under harsher movement restrictions than areas where Roma did not constitute a majority', and in Kuwait 'authorities put greater restrictions on noncitizen neighborhoods than on areas where mostly citizens live'[12] (Storer and Dawson 2020). In the UK, young men aged 18 to 34 who belong to ethnic minorities were found to be twice as likely to receive fines for breaking lockdown rules as their white counterparts.[13] From the perspective of those at the receiving end of such discriminatory practices, the narratives justifying lockdowns and other restrictions lack coherence and consistency and can have little or no resonance. No amount of rational argumentation or scientific, quantitative data brought in to support the need to abide by such measures can compensate for the immediate impact of such communities' lived experience on their decision-making process.

4.3 Transcendental Values and Conceptions of Freedom

Much of the resistance to lockdowns and other such restrictive measures during the Covid-19 crisis was informed by a specific understanding of the balance between individual freedom and social responsibility, and hence the boundaries of legitimate intervention by the state. According to Carothers and Press (2020), protests that advocated individual

[12] Non-citizens are 'a stateless Arab minority in Kuwait who were not included as citizens at the time of the country's independence or shortly thereafter' (Minority Rights Group International). They are known as *bidoon*, literally meaning 'without [nationality]'. See https://minorityrights.org/min orities/bidoon/.

[13] www.bbc.com/news/uk-53556514.

freedom over restrictive public health measures such as lockdowns and quarantines were 'generally concentrated in developed countries', including much of Europe, the USA and Canada. They were characterized by a 'wariness of science and immersion in misinformation' and 'highlight the distrust of authority that is coloring so much of global politics today'.

Bolsover (2020) identifies various understandings of freedom that underpin the debate about pandemic measures, all of which reveal a negative view of liberty as *freedom from restrictions*, with **freedom of movement** as a recurrent theme. Many anti-restriction posts considered freedom of movement as the ultimate expression of freedom, as evident in the following tweet, quoted by Bolsover (2020):

> #OpenCalifornia #opencalifornianow it's time people of the great nation of America to open your doors and not let a silly virus stop you!

Here, freedom of movement is conceived from the perspective of right-wing nationalism, which places much value on the protection of what it perceives as core American values (or, in other cases, core British values, core Chinese values, etc.). For some, like the author of the above tweet, these are transcendental values that trump any other value – or, for that matter, scientific evidence – because they are part of the core identity of those who hold them, a fundamental means by which they demonstrate that they belong to the community they have come to identify with. However, concerns have also been raised from a very different ethical perspective about how emergency measures negatively impact freedom of movement for vulnerable groups. In an article in *OpenDemocracy*, Mezzadra and Stierl (2020) argue that the 'stay at home' message is highly problematic for 'people who do not have a home and for whom self-quarantine is hardly an option, for people with disability who remain without care, and for people, mostly women, whose home is not a safe haven but the site of insecurity and domestic abuse'. The consequences of blanket restrictions on movement, moreover, are particularly serious for vulnerable groups who need to move in search of safety and whose freedom of movement was already restricted prior to the pandemic (Mezzadra and Stierl (2020)):

> Migrants embody in the harshest way the contradictions and tensions surrounding the freedom of movement and its denial today. It is not surprising that in the current climate, they tend to become one of the first targets of the most restrictive measures.

Not only are migrant populations subject to confinement measures that are legitimized by often spurious references to public health, but they are also deprived of 'this freedom to move' that for them represents 'safety from war and persecution, safety from poverty and hunger, safety from the virus'.

Like freedom of movement, the **right to religious assembly** constitutes a transcendental value for many worshippers, of all creeds. Bolsover (2020) quotes one tweet expressing frustration with what is clearly seen as interference in religious life in the USA – 'I'm tired of pastors getting arrested for having church services' – but similar sentiments have been expressed by other congregations in different parts of the world. Protestors in ultra-Orthodox Jewish neighbourhoods in Jerusalem, for instance, responded violently to police attempts to 'clear yeshiva classes and religious gatherings being held in violation of lockdown rules' in January 2021 (Hendrix and Rubin 2021). Many Iranian religious leaders resisted the closure of pilgrimage sites 'as an affront to their beliefs', and the caretakers of holy shrines refused to close them down (Iran News, February 2020).[14] In the holy city of Qom, one individual expressed his anger at restrictions on religious assembly by deliberately licking the grid of a shrine (Hendrix and Rubin 2021).

Not all worshippers, of course, and not all religious communities have questioned restrictions on religious assembly in the context of Covid-19. The rector of the All Saints' Anglican Church in the Waterloo region of Southern Ontario, Canada found it 'puzzling that religious communities have been at the forefront of the protests' (Veneza 2021). His own congregation had moved to virtual media to conduct their faith, prioritizing the need to 'care for one another' and recognizing that 'the simplest way and best way we can care for one another is to protect one another'. Moving to online services, he argued, had further allowed more people to participate who would otherwise not have been able to attend. Imam Abdul Syed of the Waterloo Mosque in the same region confirmed that his congregation, too, was 'willing to do its part to deal with the health crisis before returning to in-person worship' (Veneza 2021):

> "We want to see [the coronavirus] gone from the world," said Syed. "We want to see Canada as a safe place for everyone so, we don't want to put any lives in jeopardy."

Here we have two religious communities based in the same region, which seem to identify with the larger, national community in which they are embedded and are hence willing – indeed, feel obliged – to adhere to any measures that they believe would serve its welfare. Such wildly different responses to restrictions on religious assembly by equally devout communities reflect differences in political cultures, the degree of trust in policy makers and the medical establishment and a sense of belonging to a community that is either restricted to or is larger than their immediate religious group. They also reflect different understandings of freedom – in the latter case of worshippers in the Waterloo region, understood as freedom *to* rather than freedom *from*.

Ultra-religious groups of all creeds aside, concerns have also been voiced about the consequences of restrictions on religious assembly for vulnerable minority groups. Ekeløve-Slydal and Kvanvig (2020) report that in India lockdown rules were used by Hindu state officials to target the Muslim minority populations, and Hasan (2020) confirms that the targeting of Muslims was sanctioned at the highest levels:

> The government itself has blamed around a third of India's confirmed Covid-19 cases on a gathering held in Delhi by a conservative Muslim missionary group called the Tablighi Jamaat; one BJP minister called it a 'Talibani crime'.

In Georgia, religious assembly was allowed for Orthodox Christians during Easter but the authorities 'reacted with hostility when Muslims wanted to gather for Ramadan' (Ekeløve-Slydal and Kvanvig 2020). Such instances of structural and material incoherence in the implementation of restrictions serve to undermine trust in policy makers and the medical establishment, at the same time as strengthening the need among minority groups to demonstrate identification with their religious community rather than with the overall society in which they live.

---

[14] https://en.radiofarda.com/a/man-seen-licking-shrine-grids-despite-coronavirus-arrested-in-iran/30462926.html.

A 'Factsheet' on coronavirus issued by the United States Commission on International Religious Freedom at the start of the crisis, in March 2020, predicted the impact of restrictions on movement on various religious communities and called for addressing their concerns to ensure both respect for their human rights and efficacy of implementation of health policies (Weiner et al. 2020):

> It is important for governments to account for religious freedom concerns in their responses to COVID-19, for reasons of both legality and policy effectiveness. From a legal perspective, international law requires governments to preserve individual human rights, including religious freedom, when taking measures to protect public health even in times of crisis. From an efficacy perspective, considering religious freedom concerns can help build trust between governments and religious groups, who in past public health crises have played a critical role in delivering health interventions. Such concerns include the cancellation of large gatherings, among them religious activities, where viruses easily can spread.

Freedom of religious assembly is a particularly sensitive issue for many, whatever their creed, and efficacy of implementation in this area – as in many others – requires trust in medical advisers and policy makers. But trust is negatively impacted by perceptions of structural and material incoherence that remain unaddressed. As many have pointed out, pandemic restrictions do not distinguish between religious gatherings and other kinds of public events and do not provide a rationale for failing to do so. Writing on the UK Human Rights Blog, Keene (2020) argues:

> Ultimately, the right to practice religion is specifically protected by the ECHR [European Court of Human Rights] in a way that e.g. attending a football match is not. But overall the impression is given that worship and religious services have been considered together with other public gatherings or activities.

For Keene, this is particularly problematic because the evidence given to the UK Parliamentary Science and Technology Committee by the Chief Medical Officer and the Chief Scientific Adviser for England confirms that 'there has been at best very limited tailored analysis of the specific risk of transmission of Covid-19 in the context of religious services'.

4.4 Public Health Recommendations and the Values and Principles of Evidence-based Policy Making

This brings us to the nature of the medical evidence which has informed policy making throughout the pandemic and the values that underpin it. In the scholarly debate about mass public health measures, some have argued that the pandemic has changed the values and ground rules of evidence-based policy making. Since its emergence in the early 1990s, evidence-based medicine has been founded on the idea of transparent access to the evidence base underpinning healthcare recommendations, through systematic reviews of state-of-the-art research (Timmermans and Berg 2003). As such, medical evidence has arguably been detached from the expert and made available through texts that are accessible to everyone. According to Axe et al., authors of *The Price of Panic: How the Tyranny of Experts Turned a Pandemic into a Catastrophe* (Axe et al. 2020), the current pandemic has reversed these principles and replaced democratic access to evidence with 'a tyranny of experts' in which a 'narrow, professionally biased thinking dictates policy for everyone' (Axe et al. 2020:156), or as the authors put it in an article following the publication of their book, 'government bureaucrats with narrow expertise gained the status of infallible oracles' (Richards et al. 2020). A similar view is expressed by Norman Lewis on *Spiked*: 'The experts have set the goal, and the politicians have cast themselves in the role of their spokespeople' (Lewis 2020). This approach has allegedly not only 'mystified expertise' (Lewis 2020) but also maximized 'a certain kind of safety, to the neglect of other goods'. This is not necessarily a result of bad intentions on behalf of the experts, Richards et al. (2020) claim, but a result of their limited perspective:

> Such officials tend to think in bulk, to focus on the quantity of abstract life protected in the near term, rather than the quality of actual lives lived over the long term ... Looking for problems is a physician's job. Misdiagnosis could be considered malpractice. This makes them risk-averse and hypervigilant. They tend to respond to the worst-case scenario. But you, as a patient, have different aims. What you deem best for you, weighing costs and benefits, may not be what is best for the doctor who is treating you.

According to Richards et al. (Richards et al. 2020), the status and obscurantism of this new elite of medical expert bureaucrats made it possible to mask material and structural incoherence in their recommendations for some time in the initial stages of the pandemic:

> In downplaying the danger early on, the World Health Organization seemed to be carrying water for the regime in Beijing. ... But in March, the UN agency reversed course. WHO Director-General Tedros Adhanom Ghebreyesus pointed to a scary model from the Imperial College London, which predicted as many as 40 million people could die worldwide without draconian efforts to reduce the spread of the virus. It would be more than a month before non-experts learned that the model was little more than high tech, unreliable conjecture.

From a very different angle, the same experts have been accused of putting *too much* emphasis on the values of evidence-based medicine, especially randomized controlled trials. 'The search for perfect evidence may be the enemy of good policy', Trish Greenhalgh says in an interview with *Science*: 'As with parachutes for jumping out of airplanes, it is time to act without waiting for randomized controlled trial evidence' (Shell 2020). A paper Greenhalgh co-authored with Henry Rutter and Miranda Wolpert (Rutter et al. 2020) encourages public health experts to embrace uncertainty rather than searching for a unified evidence base:

> Even when an evidence base seems settled, different people will reach different conclusions with the same evidence. When the evidence base is at best inchoate, divergences will be greater. Unacknowledged or suppressed conflicts over knowledge can be destructive. But, if surfaced and debated, competing interpretations can help us productively to accept all options as flawed and requiring negotiation between a range of actors in the complex system.

The debate about various measures enforced to control the pandemic is thus closely linked to a debate about scientific rationality and its underlying values. The various issues and examples discussed in this chapter, moreover, clearly demonstrate that neither pro- nor anti-restriction discourses can make absolute claims to reason or rationality. Ultimately, we reiterate, arguments both in favour of and against lockdowns and other social restrictions are backed by values and normative commitments that are narratively rational even when not backed up by scientific evidence.

The Rational World Paradigm, the Narrative Paradigm and the Politics of Pharmaceutical Interventions

Scientists around the world have been rushing to create a series of Covid-19 vaccines that can keep up with the many variants attested to date. Health authorities in several countries, including the USA, UK, China and Russia, have aggressively promoted their vaccine candidates. At the same time, vaccine-hesitant members of many communities and anti-vaccine activists continue to question the entire vaccine project, and some even argue that the whole virus is a scam and part of a plot to profit from developing and selling vaccines and other treatments for many years to come. In what follows, we adopt Gust et al.'s (2005) and Browne's (2018) approach in considering vaccine hesitancy, vaccine scepticism and anti-vaccination as points along an attitudinal continuum rather than distinct attitudes that can be easily delineated. The spread of vaccine-hesitant and anti-vaccination narratives, moreover, must be understood against the backdrop of complex factors. One such factor is the growing mistrust of elites and experts, including official sources of medical knowledge and the institutions involved in producing and communicating this knowledge (Kennedy 2019). Doubts about the intentions of the World Health Organization (WHO) and the US Centers for Disease Control and Prevention, for instance, feature prominently in contemporary anti-vaccination narratives. Another factor is that concepts such as 'evidence' are increasingly questioned and redefined, even within parts of the medical establishment itself (Greenhalgh et al. 2014), and their role in the construction and dissemination of knowledge is being reassessed. These and other factors combine to weave a multiplicity of intersecting and complex narratives that circulate widely in all societies and impact the acceptance of various types of pharmaceutical interventions in general and the uptake of Covid-19 vaccines in particular.

The discussion regarding potential pharmaceutical treatments became highly politicized early on in the pandemic, especially after former President Trump officially endorsed the malaria drug hydroxychloroquine in April 2020, against clear medical advice, arguing 'I'm not a doctor. But I have common sense' (Brewster 2020). At that point there was no prospect of any vaccines on the horizon, and with many deaths reported daily in the USA and elsewhere, even well-informed doctors began to justify Mr Trump's hasty recommendation despite the absence of any scientific proof supporting the drug's efficacy or safety. Dr Joshua Rosenberg, a critical care doctor at Brooklyn Hospital Center, cited 'good reasons' for explaining Mr Trump's advocacy of the drug (*The New York Times*, reported by Collins 2020 in *Vox*):

> I certainly understand why the president is pushing it ... He's the president of the United States. He has to project hope. And when you are in a situation without hope, things go very

badly. So I'm not faulting him for pushing it even if there isn't a lot of science behind it, because it is, at this point, the best, most available option for use.

Other doctors argued that false hope can be damaging and criticized the former president and his supporters for cheerleading the drug in the absence of any proof of its efficacy (Collins 2020).

The debate about vaccines and treatments thus does not only reflect tensions between science and politics and expert and non-expert discourses. It also highlights the fact that there are divergent views within the scientific community itself on when new evidence may be ready to be put into political action, and what considerations – other than the findings of randomized controlled trials – might be brought to bear on the decision. The haste with which a solution had to be found to arrest the spread of the disease, and the pressure on the medical community to produce a miracle cure, both resulted in widespread discussions about studies drawing conclusions that are premature or even fraudulent (Kahn et al. 2020; Jiang 2020). This chapter explores the divergent arguments used in this debate and their various and complex value-laden underpinnings. It also engages with grassroots responses to the roll-out of Covid-19 vaccines as a case in point, drawing on historical parallels where relevant to explore some of the reasons (in Fisher's sense of *reasons* and *good reasons*; see Chapter 3) that inform the decisions different members of the community make about the desirability or safety of vaccines.

5.1 Structural and Material (In)coherence: Science and Public Policy under Pressure

Much of the intense debate and political bickering over Covid-19 vaccines in the early months of 2021, which revolved around the use of the Oxford–AstraZeneca (Vaxzevria) vaccine, arguably undermined public trust in the safety of all vaccines that were being rolled out around the same time. A number of governments paused the roll-out of the AstraZeneca vaccine in March and April 2021 in response to a very small number of serious cases of blood clotting (thrombosis) in patients who had received the first dose.[1] Structural and material incoherence in the public health messages and recommendations that followed from the decision by some governments to halt the roll-out of AstraZeneca triggered public anxiety and confusion regarding this specific vaccine and the vaccine programme more generally.

Following the first instances of reported blood clots in Denmark and Norway, the European Medicine Agency (EMA) declared on 11 March that 'there is currently no indication that vaccination has caused these conditions, which are not listed as side effects with this vaccine'.[2] A little less than a month later, the EMA's safety committee (PRAC)

---

[1] www.health.gov.au/news/atagi-statement-on-revised-recommendations-on-the-use-of-covid-19-vaccine-astrazeneca-17-june-2021. This does not compare unfavourably with the risks associated with the oral polio vaccine (OPV) at the start of the relevant vaccination programme in the USA in the 1950s. The risk to vaccine recipients and their contacts of developing paralysis was estimated as 1 in every 2.4 million doses of vaccine distributed. The balance eventually shifted with the gradual eradication of polio, ultimately resulting in no cases of paralysis reported despite continued use of OPV until 1997. See Malone and Hinman (2007) for further details.

[2] www.ema.europa.eu/en/news/covid-19-vaccine-astrazeneca-prac-investigating-cases-thrombo embolic-events-vaccines-benefits.

concluded that 'unusual blood clots with low blood platelets should be listed as very rare side effects of Vaxzevria (formerly COVID-19 Vaccine AstraZeneca)'.[3] In a statement intended for health professionals issued on the same date (7 April 2021), the EMA explicitly stated that '*a causal relationship* between the vaccination with Vaxzevria and the occurrence of thrombosis in combination with thrombocytopenia is considered plausible' (emphasis added).[4] An updated statement on 20 May makes no mention of the 'causal relationship' and instead presents the connection between the two as a mere observation: 'A combination of thrombosis and thrombocytopenia, in some cases accompanied by bleeding, *has been observed very rarely* following vaccination with Vaxzevria' (emphasis added).[5]

Another statement for health professionals about the safety and effectiveness of Covid-19 vaccines, this time issued by the WHO on 11 June 2021, similarly acknowledged that 'the AstraZeneca and Janssen COVID-19 vaccines have been associated with a very rare and unusual clotting syndrome involving thromboembolic events (blood clots) with thrombo-cytopenia (low blood platelet count)'.[6] However, the same document implicitly raised doubt about this conclusion: 'The overall number of reports received of blood clots in the veins or arteries (including venous thrombosis or venous thromboembolism) occurring without thrombocytopenia is no higher than the expected background population rate for the more common type of blood clots in most countries'.

Differences in conclusions, emphases and lack of transparency about the arguments informing the debate led by international and pan-national health authorities fuelled mistrust in both scientific and political institutions, and hence exacerbated vaccine hesi-tancy globally. A similar pattern of conflicting statements being released at different times pervaded vaccine recommendations at the national level. In Canada, the National Advisory Committee on Immunization (NACI) was accused of creating confusion with its updated Covid-19 statement on 3 May, recommending that Canadians less likely to contract Covid-19 should consider waiting for a Pfizer or Moderna vaccine instead of opting for what was then on offer, that being AstraZeneca.[7] This contradicted previous recommendations that encouraged Canadians to take whatever vaccine is available. In its new statement, NACI maintained that it would 'preferentially recommend authorized messenger RNA (mRNA) COVID-19 vaccines due to the excellent protection they provide and the absence of any safety signals of concern',[8] thereby indirectly creating the impression that AstraZeneca is a second-rate and potentially dangerous vaccine. A few days later, the Ontario government announced that it will no longer offer the Oxford–AstraZeneca Covid-19 vaccine as

---

[3] www.ema.europa.eu/en/news/astrazenecas-covid-19-vaccine-ema-finds-possible-link-very-rare-cases-unusual-blood-clots-low-blood.

[4] www.ema.europa.eu/en/documents/dhpc/direct-healthcare-professional-communication-dhpc-vaxzevria-previously-covid-19-vaccine-astrazeneca_en-0.pdf.

[5] www.ema.europa.eu/en/documents/dhpc/direct-healthcare-professional-communication-dhpc-vaxzevria/covid-19-vaccine-astrazeneca-risk-thrombosis-combination-thrombocytopenia-updated-information_en.pdf.

[6] www.who.int/news/item/11-06-2021-statement-for-healthcare-professionals-how-covid-19-vaccines-are-regulated-for-safety-and-effectiveness.

[7] www.cbc.ca/radio/asithappens/as-it-happens-tuesday-edition-1.6013354/naci-advice-to-wait-for-preferred-vaccine-sends-bad-message-to-essential-workers-doctor-1.6013526.

[8] www.canada.ca/content/dam/phac-aspc/documents/services/immunization/national-advisory-committee-on-immunization-naci/recommendations-use-covid-19-vaccines/summary-updated-statement-may-3-2021/NACI-summary-janssen-en.pdf.

a first dose due to the risk of rare blood clots. Prime Minister Justin Trudeau later sought to reassure Canadians that all vaccines approved for use in Canada are safe and effective by confirming the original recommendation of taking the first vaccine offered: 'Make sure you get your shot when it's your turn. We are continuing to recommend to everyone to get vaccinated as quickly as possible so we can get through this'.[9]

Similarly, the Australian Technical Advisory Group on Immunisation (ATAGI) advised that people between the ages of 16 and 59 should preferably receive Pfizer shots, while the government maintained that the same group of people can opt for AstraZeneca after consulting their doctors. On 28 June 2021, the prime minister Scott-Morrison declared in a press conference: 'the ATAGI advice talks about a preference for AstraZeneca to be available and made available to ... those over 60. But the advice does not preclude persons under 60 from getting the AstraZeneca vaccine ... So if you wish to get the AstraZeneca vaccine, then we would encourage you to ... go and have that discussion with your GP [general practitioner]'.[10] These and similar declarations led both journalists and medical experts to conclude that 'mixed messaging from the Australian government and ATAGI has created confusion – and hesitancy – about the available vaccines and their safety' (Shields 2021).

The confusion and controversies surrounding the Oxford–AstraZeneca vaccine and the importance accorded to the very rare reported cases of blood clotting also demonstrate the fundamentally anecdotal or narrative nature of medical evidence. As Rone (2021) points out in connection with the debate about AstraZeneca,

> Ultimately, science is based on empirical data and when there is not enough data, science cannot say things with certainty. When new data is available, scientists are ready to correct previous errors thus incrementing knowledge. Science has never been about absolute certainty. Nor has it pretended to be. That is its strength. But this does not sound very reassuring when one needs to take a personal decision affecting one's own health.

The inherent uncertainty of science means that the positions taken by various national and local governments can and often do rely more on narrative proximity and identification with the individual characters than on risk calculation based on numbers. The case of the Oxford–AstraZeneca vaccine thus confirms Fisher's claim that 'the operative principle of narrative rationality is identification rather than deliberation' (Fisher 1989:66). In Norway, a country with a small population and high life expectancy, the AstraZeneca vaccine was permanently suspended when five people were hospitalized for a combination of blood clots, bleeding and a low count of platelets after receiving the first dose. Three of them later died. On 15 April 2021, the Norwegian Medical Agency delivered a report to the Norwegian government that concluded the following: 'Since there are few who die from Covid-19 in Norway, the risk of dying from taking the AstraZeneca vaccine will be greater than the risk of dying from the disease, especially for younger people'.[11] The Norwegian Medical Agency also acknowledged that there are several uncertainties with this analysis: first, that the current spread of infection informing this conclusion could change; and second, that the relative death rates are difficult to determine, given that the estimation is based on numbers

[9] www.cbc.ca/news/politics/trudeau-tam-safe-effective-naci-1.6013297.
[10] www.pm.gov.au/media/virtual-press-conference-1.
[11] www.fhi.no/en/news/2021/astrazeneca-vaccine-removed-from-coronavirus-immunisation-programme-in-norw/.

from Norway and Denmark only.[12] Their conclusion was therefore not based on firm evidence alone but on 'good reasons', with several 'non-scientific' considerations taken into account. In particular, the agency's assessment ultimately focused on what is likely to 'ring true' to members of the public, as evident in its final justification for suspending the AstraZeneca vaccine: 'There is reason to believe that there is a high degree of skepticism about using the AstraZeneca vaccine in Norway and it is uncertain how many people would have accepted an offer of this vaccine now'.

It is worth noting at this point that governments and medical institutions are not the only narrators whose discourses influence public trust in specific vaccines or in vaccination in general. The high degree of scepticism acknowledged by the Norwegian Medical Agency is not triggered by the reported findings of specific trials alone but also by the impression of relative danger or safety created by a range of narratives circulating in public space, including narratives framed and reinforced by the media in different countries. Rone (2021), for instance, explains – based on her experience of being encouraged to take the vaccine on offer by German and Czech friends but actively discouraged from doing so by friends and family in Bulgaria – that Bulgarian media's emphasis on uncertainties surrounding vaccination and the fact that they provide space for narratives that undermine trust in vaccines, including anecdotal stories 'insisting a person gets much better immunity if they actually get sick', have led to a high level of scepticism in the country. For a long period at the start of the pandemic, Rone tells us, 'all Bulgarian mainstream media invited doctors who insisted that the virus is a simple flu, masks don't help, we need to reach herd immunity', whereas in countries such as the UK the media tend not to emphasize uncertainties, but rather 'the benefits of vaccinating as many people as possible, starting from the most vulnerable groups' (Rone 2021).

Speaking on the CTV Television Network in Canada. on 4 May 2021, the Chair of the National Advisory Committee on Immunization (NACI) in Canada, Dr Caroline Quach-Thanh, controversially admitted that risk cannot necessarily be calculated rationally: 'If, for instance, my sister was to get the AstraZeneca vaccine and die of a thrombosis when I know that it could have been prevented and that she's not in a high-risk area, I'm not sure I could live with it'.[13] She was later criticized for fuelling fear and hesitancy through her statement. On an epistemological level, however, her unguarded response reveals the extent to which medical discourses depend on narrative rationality but at the same time struggle to make sense of it. While trying to defend, from the point of view of scientific rationality, the NACI's decision to advise young people to wait for the preferred vaccine, she admitted – almost by a slip of the tongue – that what ultimately matters in practice is whether the decision to take or not take a specific vaccine is consistent with – speaks to – people's lived experience and its potential risk to loved ones, rather than its overall risk assessment. This is about whether a person embedded in space and time and emotionally connected to others can 'live with' a particular decision they have to make, not about assessments of risk in the disconnected and sanitized environment of the laboratory.

That all vaccines – indeed, all forms of pharmaceutical and medical interventions in general – carry a certain level of risk is not disputed by the scientific community nor by policy makers. But scientific rationality tends to weigh the benefits and dangers of this risk

---

[12] www.fhi.no/contentassets/3596efb4a1064c9f9c7c9e3f68ec481f/2021_04_14-anbefalingsnotat-oppdrag-21.pdf.
[13] www.youtube.com/watch?v=XNw-cg2ZKqI.

in the abstract, whereas narrative rationality works by weighing it in the context of a life lived with others. This explains why parents may be particularly wary of vaccination in general. As Larson (2020:5) explains, 'the timing of childhood vaccines coincides with a number of childhood infections and at a time when parents are particularly focused on the evolving development of their child, thus making associations with vaccines more believable and helping to fuel the contagion of rumors'. Similarly, early signs of autism coincidentally tend to become noticeable around the same time as the measles, mumps, and rubella (MMR) vaccine is given to children, 'when all parents are focused on first words, first steps' (Larson 2020:11). The risks that parents and other members of society associate with vaccines may thus not even be the actual risks science establishes and acknowledges, making the task of debunking them more difficult and complicated (Larson 2020:37). In what follows we will further unpack some of these complexities and explore ways in which understanding how narrative rationality works may give us better insight into how to address anxieties surrounding vaccination more effectively. But first a brief word about the role of characterological coherence in influencing public confidence in vaccines.

5.2 Characterological Coherence and Public Confidence in Vaccines

We saw in Chapter 2 that characterological coherence is assessed on the basis of the perceived reliability (or otherwise) of specific characters associated with a given story. For many, therefore, the fact that Neil Ferguson – the British public figurehead for the argument supporting a strict lockdown to arrest the spread of Covid-19 – was found to have flouted the rules of lockdown to meet his lover meant that his advice on the necessity of lockdowns could no longer be trusted. In the case of vaccines and other pharmaceutical interventions, characterological coherence seems to work in more contradictory ways that are influenced by centuries of public opposition to vaccination, and by repeated attempts on the part of governments to suppress this opposition by passing laws that make certain types of vaccines mandatory. Examples include the Vaccination Acts of 1853 and 1867 in England, which made vaccination against smallpox mandatory for infants up to 3 months old and then up to 14 years old, respectively. Alongside these legal measures, institutions representing medical practitioners also have a history of censuring doctors who act in ways that undermine specific vaccination campaigns. The most recent example at the time of writing is Dr Gerard Waters, who was suspended from the medical register by the High Court of Ireland in April 2021 for refusing to vaccinate his patients against Covid-19.[14] Dr Waters, who believed the vaccine to be 'untrustworthy and unnecessary' (Cullen 2021) and 'disagreed with how quickly the vaccines had been developed' (O'Connor 2021), described himself as a 'conscientious objector', thus invoking associations with pacifism and the Christian principle 'thou shalt not kill', used by the Quakers in particular to justify refusal of armed service in both world wars. The framing of a narrative such as Dr Waters's is important in influencing assessments of characterological coherence. In this case, powerful institutions are narrated as exercising their superior power against a principled individual who holds fast to his beliefs despite the adverse consequences to his career. This type of storyline appeals to particular values that many people hold dear, such as courage and integrity, which can provide 'good reasons' for believing dissenting rather than official, mainstream

---

[14] www.bmj.com/content/373/bmj.n987.

characters. The importance of such values in assessing characterological coherence is most evident in a much more high-profile case associated with anti-vaccination movements: that of Andrew Wakefield.

Andrew Wakefield is a former physician who was struck off the medical register by the UK's General Medical Council following the publication of a 1998 co-authored article in *The Lancet*,[15] which posited a link between the MMR vaccine and autism. He continues to campaign against vaccination in general and has become a cause célèbre for the anti-vaccination movement, 'a headliner for the vaccine-sceptic circuit' as Omer (2020) calls him in a review of *The Doctor Who Fooled the World* – an unauthorized biography of Wakefield written by Brian Deer (Deer 2020), the investigative reporter who first broke the story about the 1998 *Lancet* article. For many people, Wakefield's open censure by the medical community meant that he was no longer credible, and hence his arguments against vaccination could not be trusted. For others, as Larson (2020) points out, he became a symbol of integrity, of courage in the face of persecution, lending his claims believable whatever 'facts' are presented against them by the scientific community. For anti-vaccine advocacy groups such as Generation Rescue who saw Wakefield in this light, he was 'Nelson Mandela and Jesus Christ rolled up into one' (cited in Larson 2020:11). The Vaccine Resistance Movement (VRM) reinforces the impression of a Jesus Christ fighting persecution by raising donations 'to finance his many court cases' (Larson 2020:12). This example suggests that assessments of characterological coherence are entangled, at least in some cases, with the exercise of institutional power and our tendency to admire and respect those who stand up to it. It is no coincidence, therefore, that anti-vaccination websites such as Children's Health Defense, run by Robert F. Kennedy, Jr., feature extensive quotes from Mahatma Gandhi's prolific writings against vaccination.[16]

In the debate about Covid-19 vaccines and vaccination more generally, assessment of characterological coherence does not only apply to individuals but also to nations and institutions. Just as Bakan (2003) asked in his famous book *The Corporation*, what the personality of the corporation would be if it were a person, we all have a tendency to associate various types of institutions and governments with certain qualities, on the basis of which we become more or less trusting of their discourses. In our current context, this is particularly evident in the case of countries and institutions involved in the debate on global vaccine distribution, and more specifically, the Agreement on Trade-Related Aspects of Intellectual Property Rights (TRIPS) and its consequences for the Covid-19 response. In October 2020, India and South Africa proposed a waiver to the intellectual property (IP) regulations defined through this agreement in order to give poorer countries access to the vaccine recipes and hence facilitate local vaccine production. The waiver was supported by 62 member states of the World Trade Organization (WTO), but several wealthy countries and pan-national institutions, including the USA, the UK and the European Union, initially opposed it. While insisting that they are all committed to work with low and middle income countries to achieve 'equitable access to vaccines across the globe',[17] these key participants in the debate maintained that changing the IP rules would be unproductive, and as formulated in a statement by the UK government addressed to the TRIPS Council, would

---

[15] The article was later retracted by *The Lancet* in 2010.
[16] https://childrenshealthdefense.org/media-interviews/gandhi-words-from-100-years-ago-on-vaccination/.
[17] www.keionline.org/34275.

constitute an 'extreme measure to address an unproven problem'.[18] Dangor and Sucker (2021), members of a group of academic lawyers which included an advisor to the South African government on international relations, saw the response to the waiver as part of a more pervasive pattern of characterological incoherence that many have come to associate with wealthy countries; these tend to advocate global governance along paradoxical lines that are ultimately intended to ensure their own national interests:

> ... while committing to work with UN-led initiatives such as the Covid-19 Vaccine Global Access Facility (Covax), ostensibly aimed at equitable and science-led global vaccine distribution, the richer countries undermined such collective processes by practising vaccine nationalism – signing agreements with pharmaceutical companies to supply their own populations in a manner that reduces equitable access for others, often leading to forms of vaccine apartheid between countries ... That the rich countries, which purport to champion global governance, acted contrary to and in a manner that undermined UN-led initiatives to create global governance bodies to allocate and distribute the vaccines based on science and ethics, underscores the sentiment in much of the global south that rich countries of the north instrumentalise the institutions of global governance in ways that are only beneficial to them.

Homer (2021) offers a detailed example of the type of behaviour that underpins perceptions of characterological incoherence in relation to specific rich countries in this context:

> In June, the G7 countries pledged to donate 1 billion doses to 'poor countries', with the UK pledging 100 million of them. Yet so far, the UK has delivered only 5.1 million doses to Covax and sent just 10.3 million abroad in total. At the same time, the UK has actually taken doses from Covax that it has a right to (many other wealthy countries have waived their right to their share). In June, the same month it made its 100-million-dose pledge, the UK received 539,000 doses from Covax, more than double the doses Covax sent to Africa in the same month.

Similarly, in an analysis of the EU's response to the waiver, Engebretsen and Ottersen (2021) explain how the EU paradoxically uses 'global collaboration' as an argument against the global right to vaccine production. In claiming that 'in a global pandemic only broad and equitable access to vaccines across the globe will ensure that the public health crisis can be tackled effectively, including *in developing countries that have no production capacities*' (emphasis added),[19] the lack of production capacities in poor countries is presented as an indisputable fact. Global collaboration accordingly is assumed to consist of compensating for this lack by increasing vaccine access through means other than sharing the recipe with all nations. There is no room here for considering the possibility of mitigating the presumed lack by supporting the development of production capacities in poor countries. This logic 'leads to a paradox' some have come to associate with the character of wealthy nations: in this particular context, '[l]ack of efficiency and capacity in the health service in poor countries is used as an argument for globally defined measures, and against contributing to the development of capacity and improving efficiency by allowing these countries to develop vaccines and treatment programs themselves' (Engebretsen and Ottersen 2021).

---

[18] www.gov.uk/government/news/uk-statement-to-the-trips-council-item-15.
[19] www.keionline.org/34275.

For some, then, arguments against sharing vaccine recipes – such as 'IP protections provide incentives to companies to create new and groundbreaking technologies' (Lee and Holt 2021) – are bogus and consistent with the exploitative and dishonest character of rich countries and corporations intent on blocking the development of vaccine production capacity in poor countries. For others, it must be acknowledged, such arguments will continue to be perceived as not only rational and realistic but also as indicative of the responsible character of the governments that promote them and their laudable loyalty, above all, to their own populations. What has been negatively referred to in much of the literature and the media as 'vaccine nationalism' (Weintraub et al. 2020; Eaton 2021; Khan 2021; Lagman 2021; Mayta et al. 2021) has thus been explained by others in pragmatic terms as a case of governments like the UK's sensibly 'striking deals early because, without the upfront investment from rich countries, ... vaccine manufacturers would not be making any vaccine at risk' (Torjesen 2020). The term 'vaccine nationalism' appeared in the late spring of 2020 and 'is linked to agreements that reserve the bulk of emerging vaccines for a limited number of countries, traditionally in the developed world' (Rutschman 2020). The strategy adopted is not new – a similar pattern of rich countries hoarding vaccine production for their own populations was also evident in the case of the H1N1 flu in 2009 (popularly known as swine flu). But the strategy and the narratives that underpin and justify it are now a 'hallmark of negotiations during large-scale outbreaks of vaccine-preventable diseases' (Rutschman 2020). The feminist writer Rosebell Kagumire adopts the term 'vaccine apartheid' (rather than 'vaccine nationalism'): this has gained some currency and is used, along with hashtags such as #EndVaccineApartheid and #EndVaccineInjusticeInAfrica, to demand that immediate action be taken to alleviate acute Covid-19 vaccine shortages (Kagumire 2021). Kagumire argues that the emergence of the Omicron variant in November 2021, which was initially assumed to have originated in South Africa (see Chapter 1), revealed the colonial undertones of the policies adopted by wealthier countries. Rather than praising the South African government for its transparency and working with it to address this new source of threat, the European Union, the USA and the UK decided to impose a banket travel ban on Southern Africa and neighbouring countries. 'At the same time', Kagumire points out,

> the emergence of 'variants of concern' across the world (including Europe) and growing COVID-19 death toll among unvaccinated populations have not dissuaded the West from pursuing vaccine hoarding and vaccine nationalism policies.

By privileging some human lives over others, Western countries thus arguably prolong the pandemic and impact not just the lives and livelihoods of marginalized populations, but also of those they set out to protect.

5.3 Transcendental Values and Conceptions of Freedom

Policies adopted by governments and other institutional bodies in relation to pharmaceutical interventions such as vaccination may be seen as rational, fair and reassuring by some members of the public and as intrusive, discriminatory and oppressive by others. The issue here is not simply one of assessing the structural, material and characterological coherence of a given argument and those who advocate it, though such assessment does play a role in this as in all other contexts. How individuals respond to institutional measures such as those mandating vaccination is ultimately also informed by the transcendental values to which they subscribe and that constitute the core of narrative rationality. As Kaebnick and Gusmano (2019) put it, 'Before we can make a meaningful dent in the number of people who refuse to vaccinate their children, we have to accept that "because science" won't convince anyone. At the end of the day, it's values – beliefs about what matters, what's important, what should guide our lives and societies – that are most important'.

One such value determines our approach to the balance between personal freedom and social responsibility that we already saw play a major role in shaping responses to restrictive measures such as lockdowns and quarantines (Chapter 4). People are generally aware of the importance of balancing personal needs and convictions with those of society at large, and can steer a course that avoids direct conflict between the two under most circumstances. The more intrusive and severe the measures adopted to control individual behaviour, however, the more likely it is for increasing numbers of people to react negatively to the intrusion into their personal lives, and – importantly – into those of others, irrespective of their own position on the subject of intrusion. Hence, for instance, a January 2021 survey of potential acceptance of a Covid-19 vaccine that involved 13,426 people in 19 countries found 'a discrepancy between reported acceptance of a COVID-19 vaccine and acceptance if vaccination was mandated by one's employer'. All respondents to the survey, 'regardless of nationality' and despite marked differences in the level of vaccine acceptance across countries, 'reported that they would be less likely to accept a COVID-19 vaccine if it were mandated by employers' (Lazarus et al. 2021:226). Similarly, Reuters reported in November 2021 that almost 50% of employees at aircraft companies based in Kansas were defying the federal mandate to be vaccinated, at the risk of losing their jobs. Importantly, the head of the Machinists union district is quoted as asserting that many employees 'did not object to the vaccines as such . . . but were staunchly opposed to what they see as government meddling in personal health decisions' (Bellon and Johnson 2021). Lazarus et al. thus conclude that their finding regarding widespread rejection of mandated vaccination 'across all countries with both high and low reported vaccine acceptance proportions suggests that promoting voluntary acceptance is a better option for employers' (Lazarus et al. 2021:226).

At the same time, the more serious a threat to the smooth running of everyday life and the survival of a community, the more likely that those in charge – including governments and employers – will intervene to control individual behaviour. Nowhere is the tension between individual freedom and overall public interest more pronounced than in the fraught history of vaccination, precisely because while '[s]tanding up for rights to freedom of expression, choice, and individual dignity are all healthy characteristics of democratic societies', as Larson explains, 'contrarian views are problematic for a technology like vaccines whose success – at least for many vaccines – depends on "herd" or population cooperation to reach herd immunity' (Larson 2020:54). Whatever the justification, historical instances of mandating vaccination invariably resulted in mass protests and anger. The latest attempts to impose vaccine passports during the Covid-19 crisis is no exception (Figure 5.1).

Mandatory vaccination is a highly controversial topic whose history goes back to the middle of the nineteenth century and various national responses to the spread of smallpox at the time. As mentioned earlier, for example, vaccination against smallpox became compulsory in England in 1853 for all infants in their first three months of life, with the 1867 Act extending this requirement to age 14 and imposing severe penalties on parents who failed to vaccinate their children. Seen as a serious encroachment on civil liberties, resistance to these acts grew stronger over the years and eventually led to the

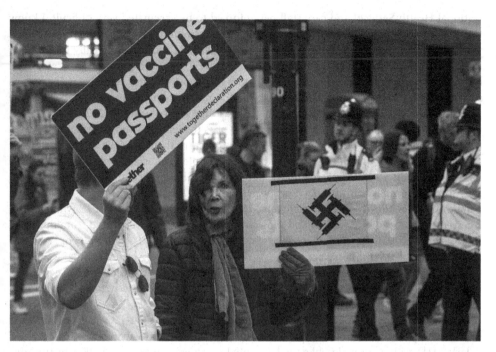

Figure 5.1 Worldwide Rally for Freedom, London, 21 November 2021. Guy Smallman / Contributor / Getty Images.

passing of the 1898 Vaccination Act, which introduced a 'conscience clause' allowing parents who had serious concerns about vaccination to obtain a certificate of exemption (Wolfe and Sharpe 2002). Interestingly, it was this Vaccination Act that introduced into English law the now widely used term 'conscientious objector', which we tend to associate with the right to refuse military conscription on grounds of freedom of conscience, thought or religious belief. It is this history, and the association of the anti-vaccination stance with the idea of challenging powerful institutions, that might explain assertions such as 'anti-vaccination is not only a belief but a *cause*' (Bruton 2020:63; emphasis in original).

Arguments against vaccination based on individual freedom can thus attract followers who are happy to be vaccinated themselves but because they 'believe in the more fundamental democratic right to choose', they see the issue from the perspective of others' right to 'dignity and respect' (Larson 2020:30). This is a case of 'I disapprove of what you say, but I will defend to the death your right to say it' – a quote often wrongly attributed to Voltaire. Even those who would not necessarily go as far as condemning mandatory vaccination or protesting against it, given the implications of vaccine hesitancy for society at large, may nevertheless feel uncomfortable with it because it encroaches on other people's autonomy. A respiratory doctor writing as 'Anonymous' in *The Guardian* in November 2021 expresses anger at those still refusing to take the vaccine, who end up on ventilators in packed intensive care units where he or she has to fight to keep them alive. Anonymous's patience, we are told, is 'wearing thin' despite accepting that a cornerstone of the way doctors protect patients' autonomy 'is the recognition that others may reasonably make decisions we may see as irrational or wrong'. And yet, the author continues, 'I find the idea of NHS [UK

National Health Service] and care staff being forced to be vaccinated very difficult. I know that it is the right outcome, but I dislike the means of bringing it about' (Anonymous 2021).

Today, governments hesitate on the whole to mandate vaccination legally in the same intrusive manner, perhaps to avoid some of the more extreme responses that strategy has historically elicited. Instead, they adopt strategies that mostly do not involve passing laws as such but nevertheless restrict the freedom of the non-vaccinated in various ways while protecting the welfare of the population at large as they see it. As of July 2021, for instance, many countries in Europe – from Greece and Cyprus to Germany and Luxembourg – have been 'obliging their residents, as well as travellers, to carry their COVID-19 passport' to be allowed entry into any indoor public spaces such as hotels, pubs and restaurants.[20] As the number of Covid-19 cases spiked and the percentage of those vaccinated remained 'shamefully low' by comparison to other European countries, Austria went further by imposing a nationwide lockdown on 15 November 2021 on anyone over the age of 12 who had not received two doses of the vaccine and those who had not recently recovered from the virus. Those who fell into one of these two categories – 'roughly 2 million people out of a population of 8.9 million', according to the Austrian Press Agency (Linnane 2021) – could only leave their homes to fulfil a small number of essential needs (Euronews 2021). Offenders, as in the case of the smallpox mandates in the mid 1800s, were to be heavily fined. A week later, Austria decided that selective lockdowns were not working, placed the whole country under stay-at-home orders, and announced that Covid-19 vaccination would become compulsory from February 2022, 'with large fines for those who refuse to be jabbed' (Clark 2021). Other countries, like the UK, opted to allow businesses and other institutions to enact their own rules. These in turn are inclined to protect their interests by enforcing various types of restrictive measures such as those Beioley et al. (2021) label 'no jab, no job' contracts when reporting that 'some companies, ranging from UK care-home operators to large multinational groups, were considering employment contracts requiring new and existing staff to have vaccinations once Britain's adult population has been offered jabs'.

This relatively less restrictive strategy can still be rejected by many on the basis of values other than that of personal freedom, including respect for personal privacy and a commitment to non-discrimination. Thus Beioley et al. (2021) go on to report that

> [m]ost employers [in the UK] are wary of any mandatory requirement for staff to be vaccinated, which would mean handling sensitive medical data, and could leave them open to legal challenges on discrimination grounds if workers refused jabs because of a religious belief, pregnancy, or a health condition that could constitute a disability.

And yet, as one NHS doctor points out, mandatory vaccination has long been widely accepted in some sectors, including medicine: 'I cannot practice medicine in this country without having mandatory vaccinations including Hepatitis B and the MMR vaccine. So why should Covid-19 be any different?' (Batt-Rawden 2021). For many, moreover, the right of individuals to decide what they do with their bodies has to be weighed against others' right to life, and for them the value of life ultimately trumps all others. If what an individual decides to do with their bodies endangers others' lives then they must live with the restrictions society has to impose on them. Especially with the spread of what was then

---

[20] www.schengenvisainfo.com/news/covid-19-health-passes-for-accessing-public-spaces-becoming-the-norm-in-eu-16-countries-implement-such-requirements/.

termed the Indian variant of Covid-19 in the spring of 2021, some have therefore argued for very extensive measures to be adopted (O'Grady 2021):

> If we don't want this Covid crisis to last forever, we need some new simple, guidelines: No jab, no job; no jab, no access to NHS healthcare; no jab, no state education for your kids. No jab, no access to pubs, restaurants, theatres, cinemas, stadiums. No jab, no entry to the UK, and much else.

5.4 Pure Bodies, Microchips and Genetically Modified Organisms

One of the recurring objections to vaccines in general, including Covid-19 vaccines, is that they are not 'natural' and as such compromise the purity of the body, a view often traced back to Gandhi's famous writings on the subject. A hero to many, Gandhi's *Guide to Health* asserts that 'vaccination is a very dirty process' (Gandhi 2016:105). Larson (2020:12) suggests that Andrew Wakefield's anti-vaccination message resonates beyond his insistence on a link between the MMR vaccine and autism. It also 'appeals to a growing constituency of naturopathic, anti-chemical, pro-nature, alternative health audiences' (Figure 5.2). A study conducted by epidemiologists and psychologists and reported in *The New York Times* in 2021 found that people who object to vaccines are 'twice as likely to care a lot about the "purity" of their bodies and their minds' (Tavernise 2021). 'My body is a temple' is thus a common refrain for many who seek exemption from vaccination on religious grounds

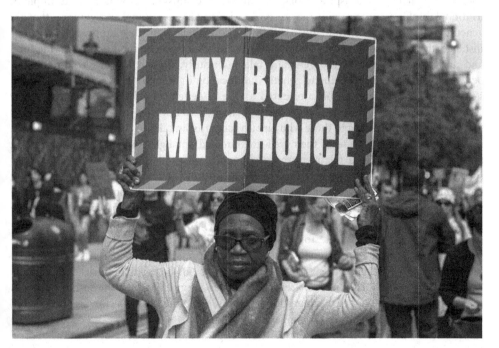

Figure 5.2 A protester in London asserts her right to making decisions concerning her body, May 2021. Copyright SOPA Images / Contributor / Getty Images.

(Stevenson 2021). The emphasis on purity is not restricted to religious groups, however. It may have its roots in religious beliefs in some cases but in others it is 'entirely secular', as in the case of 'people who care deeply about toxins in foods or in the environment' (Tavernise 2021).

A related topic concerns the use of human cells taken from aborted fetuses to test vaccines, and in some cases in their actual production. Here, it is again the question of the purity and sanctity of the human body, however underdeveloped, that informs the decision of some groups to reject specific vaccines. Thus, some US Catholic bishops described the Johnson & Johnson Covid-19 vaccine specifically as 'morally compromised' because what they called 'abortion-derived cell lines' (taken from the tissue of aborted fetuses) were used not only to test but also to develop and produce it, while others insisted that all three vaccines available in the USA (Pfizer, Moderna and Johnson & Johnson) are equally compromised for having used cell lines in the testing phase (Olmstead 2021). For other religious groups, it is not the use of fetuses but the idea that their bodies may potentially be contaminated by certain ingredients such as pork-derived gelatin – used to stabilize vaccines – that poses a problem (Milko 2020). The British Islamic Medical Association's 'Position Statement on the Moderna Covid-19 Vaccine', for example, assures its audience that '[t]he Moderna vaccination has no components of human or animal origin. The lipid nanoparticle contains cholestorol from a plant source. There is no ethanol (alcohol) in the Moderna vaccine'.[21]

A recurrent theme among some constituencies, especially on social media, is that Covid-19 vaccines contain a microchip that governments or global elites like Bill Gates intend to use for surveillance purposes (Figure 5.3), and that these intrusive measures constitute an assault not only on privacy but also on our personal health and well-being. Such beliefs are widely associated with conspiracy theories and hence dismissed outright, as an example of irrational thinking. But for many they resonate with and are as rational as arguments that are generally taken seriously by mainstream institutions, including the European Union. For instance, the concerns of activists who object to the use of genetic modification in the food and agricultural industries are generally taken seriously, despite obvious commonalities between them and those relating to genetic modification in the context of Covid-19 vaccines. Whilst mRNA vaccines can be considered a type of genetic-based therapy since they use a genetic code from Covid-19, science tells us that they do not alter our genes. But this may not sound very convincing to those who already lack trust in science, and often specifically in medical institutions because of their well-documented entanglement with politics and the neoliberal economy. Two relatively recent examples will suffice to clarify this particular source of anxiety for many people. The first is accounts of Goldman Sachs analysts weighing the economic benefits of recurring treatments vs one-shot cures and posing the question to their clients – in a report entitled 'The Genome Revolution' – 'Is curing patients a sustainable business model?' (Kim 2018). The second is ongoing concerns about the growing influence of Bill Gates's funded Institute for Health Metrics and Evaluation (IHME), based at the University of Washington. Among other sources expressing such concerns, *The Nation* published a long article in December 2020 entitled 'Are Bill Gates's billions distorting public health data' (Schwab 2020) in which several examples are given of what the author describes as the IHME's expanding and unquestioned dominion in the health sector. Reports of Bill Gates warning governments in November 2021 of smallpox terror attacks and calling for 'the formation of a new billion-dollar World Health Organisation (WHO) Pandemic Task Force'

---

[21] https://britishima.org/moderna-covid19-vaccine/.

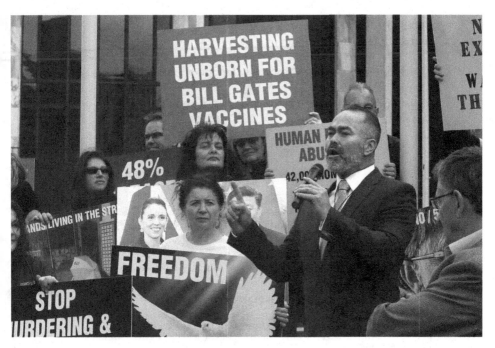

Figure 5.3 New Zealand Public Party leader Billy Te Kahika Jr speaks at a Human Rights Violations protest at Parliament on 6 August 2020. Copyright Lynn Grieveson - Newsroom / Contributor / Getty Images.

(Sky News 2021) served to further entrench the idea that global elites in general and Bill Gates in particular exercise unwarranted control over health policy.

At any rate, to go back to the issue of genetic modification and vaccine hesitancy, the similarity to gene therapy, which does involve modifying a patient's genes to cure specific diseases, and resonance with the debate about the purity of the human body that this topic evokes, both provide ample reason for many to question the wisdom of vaccination. Social media platforms abound with posts such as that shown in Figure 5.4,[22] from the Twitter feed of 'joey_di_marco', whose profile reads:

> #freedomfighter
> #antiglobalist#truthseeker#alliantie#nature#animals#thepowerofwater#ewaranon#nietsis-wathetlijkt

The idea that gene therapy is unnatural and 'anti-human', moreover, is far from new. Anti-GMO activists have drawn since the late 1980s on narratives that link GMOs (genetically modified organisms) with pollution, contamination or monstrousness (Schurman and Munro 2009). Similar narratives have also been used by politicians, especially in Europe, where the legislation on GMOs is particularly restrictive. As Christiansen et al. (2019) have pointed out, the restrictive rules imposed on GMOs are fundamentally based on the value of naturalness, since the organisms covered by the legislation are those 'in which the genetic material has been altered in a way that does not

---

[22] https://twitter.com/JongheDirk/status/1454504541702049795.

joey_di_marco @JongheDirk · Oct 30 •••
Just a shot of truth.

Check out who's exempt from this depopulation death jab. 😂 🔫

Btw, It is not a vaccine it's a death shot, a **gene therapy** that alters human dna making trans-human.

EXEMPT

All of US Congress plus all Congressional staff, House and the Senate. That's a lot of people.

6,000 White House employees.

2,500 Pfizer, 1,500 Moderna, and 120,000 Johnson and Johnson employees.

15,000 CDC and 14,000 FDA employees.

300,000 Chinese students in this country [USA].

How many of them are PLA, CCP? 85 to 90% I can tell you that.

2 million illegal aliens exempted. They don't have to get the shot.

"the rest of us, must get injected or lose our job"

OBVIOUSLY THE ABOVE SPECIAL PEOPLE AIM TO AVOID THE JAB.......WHY? MIGHT THE VACCINE BE A SECRET CAUSE OF MASS DEATH?

Figure 5.4 Post from the Twitter Feed of Joey di Marco, 30 October 2021

occur naturally by mating and/or natural recombination', according to the European Commission's archived page on biotechnology.[23] In a blog post on *The Daily Beast* that questions this rationality and the values that underpin it, Anslow (2021) thus concludes that '[i]n this pandemic anti-vaxxers didn't need to discredit 200 years of vaccine efficacy, or explain away scientific consensus. They just needed to sow doubt about emerging biotechnologies, a job that had already been largely done for them by the press and politicians. Biotechnophobia was already endemic'.

Anslow's critique of what he sees as the structurally incoherent attitudes of European politicians with regard to gene engineering is echoed by Brooks (2021), an agricultural economist, who argues in a blog post on Open Access Government that European politicians show inconsistency when they queue up to praise the breakthroughs of the new vaccines:

> These vaccines use the very same techniques of genetic modification (GM) or gene editing (GE) that most European politicians have spent the last 25 years preventing their citizens and farmers from having access to for the production and consumption of food, feed and fibre crops and which so-called environmental advocacy groups have opposed unequivocally.
>
> If these politicians and advocacy groups were being consistent with their past behaviour, they would be vigorously campaigning against these vaccines' approval and publicly stating that they personally will not be using them.

---

[23] https://ec.europa.eu/environment/archives/biotechnology/index_en.htm.

5.5 Resonance, Lived Experience and Trust

As mentioned earlier in this chapter and Chapter 3, and discussed in detail in Chapter 2, Fisher considers identification as the operative principle of the narrative paradigm (Fisher 1987:66). A story, according to him, 'not only says something about the world, it also implies an audience, persons who conceive of themselves in very specific ways' (Fisher 1987:75), and it is only when the story resonates with the 'self-conception' of this audience that they can and will accept it as true. Conversely, 'if a story denies a person's self-conception, it does not matter what it says about the world' (Fisher 1987:75) – it will not resonate. In order to appeal to 'good reasons' and 'ring true' for their audience, stories must thus create resonance.

What constitutes truth is ultimately a matter of trust, and that can override even direct personal experience, in this case of the symptoms of disease. For some, like Dr Samantha Batt-Rawden, first-hand experience of the disease should be enough to convince people that they need to be vaccinated (Batt-Rawden 2021):

> I've seen first hand the damage the virus can do. I've watched it rip through whole families after they had been mixing at Christmas. Whole generations – gone. If you had seen what I have, you would be first in line for the vaccine too.

And yet, a recent study that attempted to establish what factors determine acceptance rates of Covid-19 vaccines surprisingly found that those 'who reported COVID-19 sickness in themselves or family members were no more likely to respond positively' to the question of whether they would accept vaccination than those who hadn't experienced the illness first hand. At the same time, those 'who said that they trusted their government were more likely to accept a vaccine than those who said that they did not' (Lazarus et al. 2021:226). Indeed, countries where levels of acceptance were above 80% 'tended to be Asian nations with strong trust in central governments (China, South Korea and Singapore)' (Lazarus et al. 2021:226). In France, by contrast, confidence in medical science has declined following various scandals involving the government and drug companies. 'The most famous of these', according to a *Foreign Policy* report which suggests this to be the 'real reason France is skeptical of vaccines', concerns 'the diabetes drug Mediator, which was marketed as a weight loss pill and has been linked to the deaths of as many as 2,000 people' (Chabal 2021). In many cases, therefore, lack of trust in Covid-19 vaccines among particular populations has less to do with the vaccines themselves than with a lack of trust in the governments, healthcare systems and pharmaceutical companies that promote them (Figure 5.5). As pointed out in a 2019 editorial in *The Lancet Infectious Disease*,[24] this distrust is far from irrational, even by the traditional view of rationality that we question here. The editorial argues, for instance, that reluctance to seek proper care during the Ebola outbreak in the Democratic Republic of Congo and the uncontrolled transmission that it provoked was due to a deep distrust in the government that followed from years of neglect and corruption. It concludes that 'a belief that vaccines cause autism or that Ebola is a government ploy likely has as much to do with wider grievances and distrust of authority as with the specifics of the scientific evidence and education'. Stories of abuse of authority on the part of governments and other institutions ring true because they resonate with people's previous experiences or with stories they have been told by their friends and family – those with whom they identify and can trust. And they have a long history: John Gibbs's 1854 treaty against compulsory

---

[24] www.thelancet.com/journals/laninf/article/PIIS1473-3099(19)30128-8/fulltext.

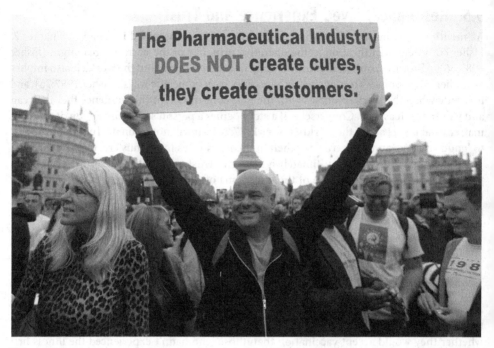

Figure 5.5 Anti-lockdown and anti-vaccine protest in London July 2021. Copyright Anadolu Agency / Contributor / Getty Images.

vaccination, *Our Medical Liberties*, complained – among other things – that the Vaccination Act of 1853 'was written to benefit the medical trade', not the populace (PopMatters 2020).

Jamison et al. (2019) explored the levels of trust in pharmaceutical companies and government agencies that promote them among White and African American adults, focusing on the influenza vaccine. The study shows that pharmaceutical companies are widely distrusted: 'Individuals suspect that the motives governing these institutions are more aligned to generating profit than serving the public good and that pharmaceutical profits corrupt the entire healthcare industry' (Jamison et al. 2019:92). Perhaps most importantly, the study also confirms that the racialized history of American healthcare continues to impact institutional trust among African Americans. Many researchers have documented ways in which the African American population is treated differently from White patients in the USA. Annual reports from the Agency for Healthcare Research and Quality show that 40% of the measured health quality outcomes were more negative for African Americans than the White population (AHRQ 2018). Profound distrust in the motives of health institutions among the Black population is also rooted in history. An extreme example of the kind of systemic racism this part of the population has suffered is the so-called Tuskegee Syphilis Study, which was conducted between 1932 and 1972 by the United States Public Health Service and the Centers for Disease Control and Prevention on a group of nearly 400 African Americans with syphilis. Participants were told that they were receiving free medical care; in fact, they were merely being observed for a study of untreated syphilis. Dozens died as a result (Kum 2020). In Pakistan, one of the few countries where polio has not yet been eradicated and where those attempting to administer the polio vaccine are often violently attacked, 49% of the population are reported to refuse Covid-19 vaccination (Siddiqui

2021). This is not difficult to understand given that while hunting for Osama Bin Laden as recently as 2011 the US Central Intelligence Agency organized a fake vaccination programme against hepatitis B, beginning with poorer neighbourhoods which were more likely to be hiding their target (Siddiqui 2021), and used that campaign as a cover to collect DNA samples that eventually confirmed his location (Carr 2021).

Recent studies have shown that Covid-19 vaccine hesitancy is particularly prevalent amongst Black, Asian and minority ethnic (BAME) populations, and that some of this hesitancy is 'likely grounded in a long history of structurally racist systems which have led to health inequalities and injustices' (Forman et al. 2021). Even though a given Black person may never have been subjected to the kind of extreme racism described in these narratives, they will still be apprehensive about health authorities and institutions because they will see themselves as part of that group and hence a potential target of discrimination. Morgan (2021) shows how this kind of reasoning influenced the response among people from BAME groups when the medical authorities proposed starting the vaccine roll-out with the most vulnerable communities during the first wave of the pandemic:

> This caused concern among these communities, because they are not normally at the front of the queue when it comes to the best medical treatments, particularly those in lower socioeconomic classes. Some people began to speculate that it was because it was an experimental vaccine and Black people were being used as guinea pigs.

Morgan (2021) concludes that for some, 'this will have triggered alarm bells and brought up the many historical examples of Black people being used for experimental or unethical medical treatments'.

Forman et al. report that numerous surveys conducted in the UK, USA and several other countries found that respondents from historically marginalized groups, such as the BAME community, 'are less likely to accept the [Covid-19] vaccine compared to White counterparts' (Forman et al. 2021:561); they suggest that this is at least due to 'distrust of the medical profession' that is 'grounded in a long history of structurally racist systems which have led to health inequalities and injustices' (Forman et al. 2021:561). Native Americans are similarly reported to have grave concerns about vaccination. These concerns are rooted in a parallel history of discrimination that featured, among other things, the sterilization of at least 25% of all Native women of childbearing age in the 1970s (Theobald 2019). No wonder, with such a history, that resistance against polio vaccines which extended into an 11-months boycott in Nigeria was fuelled by rumours that 'vaccines from the West were sterilizing children, particularly in light of the post-911 war on terrorism interpreted as a war on Muslims' (Larson 2020:xxx). Israel eventually admitted in 2013 that it had been 'sterilizing' Jewish immigrants from Ethiopia, without their knowledge or consent, by injecting them every three months with Depo-Provera, a highly effective and long-lasting contraceptive (Dawber 2013). The women thought they were being inoculated. Larson (2020) confirms that there is a persistent association of vaccines in general with attempts to sterilize various populations, although the vaccine against tetanus tends to cause more apprehension given that it focuses primarily on girls and pregnant women.

The obvious overlap among the various issues raised throughout this chapter aside, what they all demonstrate is that our decision to trust or mistrust a given source of evidence is guided by what we have called, following Fisher, *narrative rationality*. It is narrative rationality – rather than scientific 'proof' – that determines whether or not the evidence itself is accepted as reliable and acted upon accordingly. The argument at the end of the day is not between science and heresy, or rational human beings and conspiracy theorists, but between trust and non-trust, between identification and non-identification, in the course of a complex life lived with diverse others.

Objectivist vs Praxial Knowledge: Towards a Model of Situated Epistemologies and Narrative Identification

Throughout this book, we have argued that a turn to narrative – specifically, to a modified and extended version of Fisher's narrative paradigm – can offer new insights into various phenomena that continue to hinder effective healthcare communication. This argument is developed against the backdrop of the growing hegemony of evidence-based medicine (EBM) since the turn of the century and the many challenges it has faced with the spread of Covid-19 since the end of 2019. In medicine and healthcare, the orthodox version of the EBM paradigm has generally contributed to promoting an understanding of evidence as a singular phenomenon that can be ranked on a fixed scale (the so called evidence pyramid; see Chapter 1 for details), with simple observational methods at the bottom and – moving towards the top – increasingly rigorous methodologies, notably randomized controlled trials (RCTs) and systematic reviews of such trials. The basic idea is that as long as allocations to the intervention group and the control group are double masked, RCTs are less likely to yield biased results than other types of research designs. Inherent in this assumption is the view that truth is universal and will eventually emerge once all sources of bias are eliminated. EBM researchers therefore invest in developing critical appraisal tools and checklists to evaluate whether research evidence can be considered valid, unbiased and reliable.[1] The dominance of EBM has been accompanied more recently by a growing tyranny of metrics in all areas of social life, including healthcare and health policy (Muller 2018) – especially in terms of modelling during the Covid-19 crisis. Alongside narrow understandings of evidence as defined by some of the most eager proponents of EBM, over-reliance on metrics and modelling has exacerbated an already problematic divide between traditional scientific rationality and people's lived experience. This divide, we believe, is unsustainable. One way in which it can be bridged involves appealing to our innate capacity to make sense of happenings by embedding them within narratives we can assess and act upon. Without dismissing the importance and worth of the type of knowledge produced in scientific and medical laboratories, we would therefore agree with Pabst (2021:86) that '[t]ransformative policies' must draw on the best available evidence but their success will ultimately 'depend on the persuasive power of the underlying narrative'.

In making this assertion our intention is not to devalue rationality or scientific evidence. As we explain in more detail below, our argument is that rationality itself is born out of a prerational experience, and hence the epistemological standards by which science arrives at and assesses knowledge 'are built on a foundation that they cannot themselves account for' (Qvortrup and Nielsen 2019:157). In principle, at least in its original formulation, the narrative paradigm does not dismiss traditional rationality or the value of scientific

---

[1] https://cebma.org/resources-and-tools/what-is-critical-appraisal/.

evidence, although McGee and Nelson (1985), among others, have criticized Fisher for creating an unhelpful dichotomy by pitting the rational world paradigm against the narrative paradigm. Warnick (1987:175) argues that Fisher's attitude changed over time, and that whatever his original intentions, his writings gradually implied a clear hierarchy between traditional and narrative rationality. She also criticizes Fisher for equating traditional rationality with one of its 'lesser forms', namely, 'technical rationality possessed by experts who seek to close off discussion and exclude the public from making decisions on issues of social and moral concern'. While sharing Fisher's 'commitment to communities who reason through stories', McGee and Nelson (1985:140) likewise insist that he paints a 'misleading portrait of the place of experts in public affairs'. Be that as it may: our own revised version of the narrative paradigm treats narration 'as a facet of rationality' (Stache 2018:576). Rather than assessing a particular account of some aspect of the world on the basis of an alleged universal rationality, as the canonical EBM paradigm presupposes, the version of narrative theory we adopt in this book recognizes variation in the cultural, historical and social definitions of rationality and further suggests that we ultimately assess competing narratives of the same event on the basis of the values we believe each encodes. Similarly, but from a different angle, Stengers (2002) has argued that the struggle to define a universal rationality or evidence base beyond political differences is not only impossible but counterproductive. Evidence becomes evidence 'not because it has been proven by empirical science . . . but because it has become a crossroads for heterogeneous practices, each with different interests, each of which has required the phenomena in question to be able to relate reliably to their questions and interests' (Stengers (2002):1; our translation from French). According to Stengers, bias is therefore not necessarily a negative concept; indeed, it is a prerequisite for the production of evidence. Wieringa et al. (2018b:933) further argue that there is not one but at least two different forms of bias involved in evidence-based decisions:

> When viewed from the perspective of the ideal limit theorem, bias is viewed negatively and unproductively as anything that distorts the comparisons between groups. Thus defined, bias can potentially be eliminated using technical procedures and checklists, but bias can also be defined in terms of a value-driven perspective on what is worth studying or taking into account. This kind of bias cannot be eliminated. It is unavoidable – and potentially productive and even necessary. Indeed, it could be argued that without bias, there would not be any truths at all.

In what follows, we take Fisher's narrative paradigm as a point of departure, revisit its main weaknesses (including some we discussed in earlier chapters) and draw on a number of complementary theoretical strands to address its limitations. The aim is to outline a more inclusive and socially responsive model for assessing medical knowledge and dealing with sources of controversy around health issues such as Covid-19.

6.1 Limitations of Fisher's Narrative Paradigm

Putting aside reservations about the rigidity of Fisher's dichotomy and the version of traditional rationality he assumes, the various controversies analyzed in this book demonstrate how the logic of good reasons often clashes with the rational world logic of science; some of the more extreme versions of the latter claim to have universal validity independently of the way different people experience the world. We have seen, for instance, that many in the Black, Asian and minority ethnic community have been hesitant to wear a mask in public because of the racist fears it evokes and their negative experience with law-enforcement institutions in countries such as the United States (Chapter 3). Even vaccine hesitancy can be explained with recourse to the logic of good reasons rather than being dismissed by appeals to abstract, decontextualized traditional standards of rational thinking (Chapter 5).

At the same time, Fisher's narrative paradigm is not without its more serious limitations, which have to be addressed in order to render it more productive and more amenable to being complemented with other approaches (see Section 6.2 below). One such limitation is that in asserting that stories not already familiar to and believed by an audience are unlikely to resonate with them, the narrative paradigm rests on an unhelpful tautology that fails to explain how we come to subscribe to certain narratives rather than others in the first place. The concept of narrative accrual, borrowed from Bruner (1991) and further expanded in Baker (2006), was introduced briefly in Chapter 3 as a corrective to this tautology. It suggests that we come to believe in certain narratives and the values they promote through repeated exposure to specific ways of making sense of the world. The values that underpin our decision making are not produced in a laboratory and are not arrived at by applying any logical formulae. They evolve through a long and complex process of socialization (i.e. of narrative accrual) that may span centuries and generations rather than merely years or decades, with powerful institutions such as the media, religious organizations, the family and educational systems playing a major role in this process. Narrative accrual normalizes certain accounts of the world and masks others from view. As Baker (2006:11) explains, the normalized accounts it sanctions eventually 'come to be perceived as self-evident, benign, uncontestable and non-controversial', however morally and practically untenable they may seem to those not socialized into the same set of narratives. This is borne out by the fact that earlier generations have largely seen little wrong with slavery, with the burning of those suspected of witchcraft or with policies and customs that marginalized women and castigated gays in ways that strike us as barbaric today. It is precisely this normalizing effect of narratives that requires us to complement the narrative paradigm with an approach capable of accommodating stories that 'contest social reality' (Baker 2006:163), that challenge rather than simply reinforce existing beliefs. This brings us to another, more serious limitation of the narrative paradigm as elaborated by Fisher.

Fisher's tautology has a more serious flaw than failing to explain how we come to believe in specific stories. Its emphasis on resonance may imply that we can only entertain stories that reinforce our existing beliefs and values; if taken at face value, this would condemn us to live within the limits of our current moral imagination (Kirkwood 1992:34). As Morooka (2002) argues, by 'appealing to the common sense of audiences', that is, to their existing beliefs, 'storytellers may degenerate into what Bourdieu calls doxosphers who do little more than reinforce the *doxic* submission to the social world'. In perpetuating or appearing to perpetuate the status quo, the narrative paradigm also fails to account for the dynamic movement of narratives as they evolve, multiply, splinter, are repeatedly contested and continually recast in all areas of social life. These dynamics can only be captured by attending to the tension between the normalizing, self-perpetuating aspect of narrativity and the simultaneous ability of stories to disclose the world in original ways (Sadler 2022). Any ethically responsible theory of narrative must be able to accommodate stories that challenge rather than reinforce our established beliefs and biases. Kirkwood (1992) thus calls for a rhetoric of possibility as a central component of moral argument, for acknowledging that rhetors have a responsibility not only to attend to (and reinforce) an audience's existing beliefs but also to disclose new ways of understanding the world to them. It is possible to do so, we believe, by revisiting the interplay of fidelity and probability. The two dimensions of evaluation are conceived as mutually interdependent, which means that the decision of whether an experience has 'truth qualities' and rings true to the reader, whether it has fidelity, cannot be made independently of the internal logic of the story (its narrative probability).

Fidelity does not require the audience to actually *share* the experiences of protagonists such as Black populations and their reasons for a lack of trust in health authorities during the pandemic. It merely requires that these protagonists' experiences appear to the audience to be 'true to life – in principle' (Fisher 1987:176). Hence our ability to empathize with characters in a film or novel, which merely requires that we can imagine ourselves in their position despite believing the story to be fictional. The story of Frankenstein can likewise be 'true to life – in principle' in the sense of accounting for experiences that seem real or credible 'given the universe in which the characters live and the logic of their story' (Fisher 1987:176). It is important in this context to note that Fisher's notion of fidelity is based on a rhetorical concept of truth, as truthfulness in the eyes of an audience, meaning that the truth qualities of a story are understood to be a product of the rhetorical situation rather than of correspondence with an external reality. Hence, it is possible to acknowledge the truth qualities of a given story, provided it is coherent within its own universe, without accepting it as true in any objective sense. This tension between probability and fidelity, we believe, can be exploited to provide an opening for an audience to acknowledge the truth qualities of a new and unknown universe. In other words, the audience can be encouraged to imagine themselves as characters in a story and to accept that, had they been these characters, their experiences would probably have been similar (Fisher 1987). In this lies a possibility for stories to challenge our established world views and introduce an alternative universe. Although the fidelity of a story requires that it resonates with our experiences, a carefully crafted story can also move us to new and unexpected places. The tension between normalization and disclosure, emphasized by Sadler (2022), is thus potentially present in Fisher's version of the narrative paradigm, contrary to what some of his critics have claimed.

The indirect implication in the narrative paradigm that effective stories 'cannot and perhaps should not exceed people's values and beliefs, whether or not these are admirable or accurate' (Kirkwood 1992:30) has consequences for the way we approach medical communication and policy making. If taken at face value, it may suggest, for instance, that policy making could or should be reduced to adjusting stories to people's existing beliefs rather than adjusting people's beliefs to new, evolving stories. We reject such implications, whether or not they are warranted by or intended in Fisher's approach to narrativity. Instead, we would reiterate that rhetors – including policy makers and those working in the field of healthcare communication – have a moral duty to expand the horizons of their audience beyond their current beliefs and values. This requires acknowledging that incoherence and contradiction, which are considered problematic in the narrative paradigm, can sometimes offer 'potential entry points for novel ideas and values into the auditor's belief system' (Stroud 2002:387). Recognizing inconsistencies and contradictions as potentially productive and revealing of different ways of understanding an issue in turn requires more engagement with cultural variation than can be found in Fisher's writings. As Stroud (2002:390, n4) argues, the emphasis on coherence and lack of contradiction in Fisher is itself a product of his focus on a Western context (including 'modern American political rhetoric, modern American literary texts, and a Greek philosophical dialogue from Plato') in which consistency is highly valued. In multivalent texts such as the Indian *Avadhoota Gita* and *Devi Gita*, by contrast, lack of consistency is not necessarily problematic: these narratives articulate contradictory value structures 'in such a way as to force the audience to reconstruct how they interact with and what the text "means"' (Stroud 2002:389). When connected to familiar notions, the confrontation with foreign narratives and values can trigger new insights and enable change. In such cases, it is 'the auditor that rings true to new ideas and values within a foreign narrative' (Stroud 2002:389). Stroud therefore suggests redefining narrative fidelity as 'whether or not a story "rings true" with the values that an auditor holds *or potentially could hold*, given a coherent reconstruction of the narrative in question' (Stroud 2002:389; emphasis added).

A related critique concerns some implications of Fisher's assertion that narrative rationality 'is a capacity we all have' (Fisher 1984:9) and, more specifically, that 'the people' have a natural capacity to judge stories that are told for or about them. They can misjudge stories; they can be wrong, but so can experts and elites. The problem is that Fisher goes on to argue – following Aristotle – that 'the people' 'have a natural tendency to prefer the true and the just' (Fisher 1984:9). In other words, from a narrative paradigm perspective, we all 'have a natural tendency to prefer the true and the just' *because* we all possess the capacity of narrative rationality. But as Warnick (1987) contends, such assertions ignore the widespread success of Nazi propaganda and a host of other highly unjust and destructive narratives that plague our societies. Such stock political narratives (Bennett and Edelman 1985) persuade – they have resonance – precisely because they offer people attractive scapegoats that absolve them of responsibility for various social ills and allow them to maintain the 'best conception' of themselves and their immediate communities. In other words, they rank high on narrative fidelity. Warnick thus criticizes Fisher for acknowledging that 'the people' can be wrong but remaining silent 'on the question of how they can avoid being deluded, given the absence of traditional rationality' (Warnick 1987:177). Rowland (1987:272) similarly argues that traditional rationality need not be elitist; at the same time, 'narrative modes of argument are not necessarily democratic. There is nothing inherent in storytelling that guarantees that the elites will not control a society'.

We suggest that some of the limitations in Fisher's narrative paradigm can be addressed by acknowledging the importance of opening people's minds to 'creative possibilities' that they may not be alert to, and by constructing narratives that 'provoke intellectual struggle . . . and the creation of a more workable human order' (Bennett and Edelman 1985:162; Baker 2006). To sensitize audiences to the self-perpetuating, conservative aspect of narrativity, it is important to enhance their critical skills; to encourage them to adopt a critical stance towards all narratives rather than accept dominant conceptions that circulate in their environment without scrutiny. This is, after all, the ultimate goal of education, especially at university level.

6.2 Revisiting and Extending the Narrative Paradigm

Public health is strongly linked to communication and persuasion, in that efforts to change behaviour are necessarily communicative acts. In order to design and communicate effective public health measures, we propose, health authorities must acknowledge and engage with stories like those we have documented in earlier chapters. The concerns of those who object to various restrictions such as wearing face masks or who are vaccine hesitant can only be addressed and contested by understanding and engaging with the logics of the stories to which they subscribe. Despite the limitations of the narrative paradigm as acknowledged above, and with the various caveats we have outlined to temper its basic dichotomy (traditional vs narrative rationality), our claim remains that public health discourse is too concerned with facts and not sufficiently concerned with stories. The crucial question for the success of health policy interventions is not only 'what are the facts' but 'how do these facts make sense to people, and why'. This does not mean that establishing and communicating scientific facts is not essential to successful public health work. Rather, it means that we do not get anywhere with science unless it makes sense to people. Therefore, scientific facts need to be presented in a manner that either resonates with people's current values and experiences or is capable of alerting them to new possibilities they can potentially make sense of and buy into. Facts cannot make sense in a vacuum: they only make sense as stories that reinforce or productively challenge the narratives that make up our existing moral universe.

Epistemologically, we may follow Fisher in distinguishing between information, knowledge and wisdom (Fisher 1995:172–173). Information, or what Fisher also refers to as 'objectivist knowledge' (Fisher 1995:173), is often linked to the idea of data as self-interpreting 'facts', in contrast to 'knowledge', which is assumed to have 'semantic value' and thus to require interpretation (Fisher 1995:173). Wisdom, finally, is about 'knowing whether' and is fundamentally concerned with values and 'life as it ought to be lived' (Fisher 1987:73). Facts are the cornerstone of the rational world paradigm, which proceeds by considering 'whether the statements in a message that purport to be "facts" are indeed "facts"' (Baker 2006:152). The narrative paradigm, on the other hand, considers all facts to be value-laden and assumes that assessing whatever is presented as fact always involves considering 'the explicit or implicit values embedded in a message' (Baker 2006:153). All facts then become knowledge that has to be interpreted and require wisdom to be evaluated and acted upon.

Writing in *The Conversation* in July 2021, Manuel León Urrutia draws attention to how Covid-19 data have proved to be complex and changeable. As an expert in data literacy, he reflects on how the visibility of data 'has assumed a central role in determining the degree of society's freedom since March 2020' (Urrutia 2021). Highly specialist statistical jargon and data visualizations now pervade public discourse about the pandemic. But as the author argues, increased knowledge of specialized terms such as 'flattening the curve' do not necessarily contribute to better understanding, and even less to increased consensus about the need for various types of intervention. On the contrary, 'this data deluge can contribute to the polarisation of public discourse' rather than resolving controversies. Although data are 'supposed to be objective and empirical', Urrutia argues, they 'assumed a political, subjective hue during the pandemic'. This is understandable given that people can only make sense of data by incorporating it into larger narratives of the pandemic. It means that rather than trying to resolve controversies by providing more data, which is the standard public health approach, health authorities need to engage more actively with people's values and experiences – that means, with the stories that circulate in our communities.

As discussed in Chapter 2, Fisher stresses that while the philosophical ground of the rational world paradigm is epistemology, that of the narrative paradigm is ontology (Fisher 1987:65). Stroud also acknowledges the ontological nature of Fisher's project, pointing out that narration, according to Fisher, 'is fundamentally linked to the ontology and practices of human society' (Stroud 2002:372). The narrative paradigm is concerned with the primary mode of being in the world, with the way in which we instinctively and pre-reflectively embed an experience within a story or the set of stories that constitute our world in order to make sense of it. To foreground the ontological grounds of the narrative paradigm, Qvortrup and Nielsen (2019) suggest exploring an implicit but less developed part of Fisher's theory: the concept of *dwelling*. Fisher (Fisher 1987:94) refers specifically to this concept and to his indebtedness to Heidegger:

> Particularly helpful to me is Heidegger's view that 'man is a thinking, that is, a mediating being'. This concept was put forth as an antithesis to the idea that 'man' is, or should be always, a 'calculative thinker, a person who "computes"' – weighs, measures and counts – possibilities, benefits and outcomes but does not 'contemplate the meaning which reigns in everything that is' . . . In another essay, Heidegger celebrates a line from a poem by Friedrich Hölderlin: 'Poetically Man Dwells'. I would alter the line to read: 'Narratively Persons Dwell'.

By introducing *homo narrans* as the root metaphor to describe the primary nature of human beings, Fisher suggests that 'symbols are created and communicated ultimately as stories meant to give order to human experience and to induce others to *dwell* in them in order to establish ways of living in common' (Fisher 1987:63; emphasis added). Stories are not merely modes of discourse or objects of inquiry but modes of living; we do not *use* narratives as we *use* an argument to support a predefined rational purpose. We live by and within stories in the sense that our rationality, our purposes and the arguments we use to support them are always already framed by and embedded in a narrative (or a range of narratives) within which they make sense. Fisher further insists that narration is not restricted to the mythical or fictional aspects of human communication. Similarly to Heidegger, he refutes interpretations of logos as 'reason, judgement, concept, definition, ground'; these interpretations build on an epistemology that regards truth as a question of 'accordance' or 'correspondence' (Qvortrup and Nielsen 2019:147). Instead, Fisher evokes the 'original conception of logos', which he traces back to Isocrates, for whom logos was consubstantial with discourse. Discourse is not understood here simply as the form that an expression takes but is rather assumed to encompass 'outward and inward thought' as well as 'reason, feeling and imagination' – an understanding Fisher traces back to pre-Socratic times, when a clear distinction between logos and mythos had not yet been drawn (Fisher 1987:6). At that early stage, all communicative behaviour was deemed rational, though in a variety of different ways, suggesting that it is not only philosophical and technical discourses that exhibit logos, but rhetoric and poetics too (Fisher 1987:24). Fisher proposes a return to this early conception of logos and to treating narration not as distinct from but as a type of logic, a fundamental interpretation of the world that is articulated through all forms of discourse and inhabits our thinking.

Narration, then, is an expression of a 'pre-thematic' and pre-reflective relation to the world, in the sense that 'access to reality is not to be established; it is always already established because the primary mode of being in the world is to engage with it or to dwell in it' (Qvortrup and Nielsen 2019:147). The problem with the rational world paradigm is that it tends to reduce the *ontological* (ways of 'being in the world') to the *ontic* ('being as brute facts') and practical problems to scientific ones (Heidegger 2010; Sadler 2022). The overall aim of phenomenology, as outlined by Heidegger and adopted by Fisher, is to 'establish a method that transcends what is known or given to modern man, science, or history of philosophy' (Qvortrup and Nielsen 2019:146). As such, the narrative paradigm is an attempt to capture the 'basic experience of the world of which science is the second-order expression' and on which science is established (Merleau-Ponty 1962:ix; Qvortrup and Nielsen 2019:148). At the same time, and equally important, it is a response to the phenomenological call to 'de-structure' or deconstruct the history of ontology by making the fundamental structures of this tradition explicit. Fisher's ambition, as we recall, was not solely to acknowledge the role of narratives in making sense of the world, but also to provide a framework that can explain how we assess narratives in order to decide whether or not we should adhere to them as a basis for belief and action (Fisher 1987). While Fisher presented his project as descriptive, he has been criticized for borrowing from the rational world paradigm when introducing narrative rationality as a normative standard. Conceptualizing the narrative paradigm from the perspective of narrative dwelling partly addresses this ambiguity by insisting on the fundamentally *situated* character of narrative rationality, which 'follow[s] the internal flows of a given narrative toward its goals rather than a detached evaluation of its external traits' (Qvortrup and Nielsen 2019:152). The truth qualities of a given story can never be assessed from a safe place outside and beyond the story itself, through reason as such, because reason always already *dwells* within a story. It follows that a story may be evaluated based not only on the situated principles defined within the story itself, but also with reference to the situated principles and values of the stories that its audience brings into the assessment. The latter may resonate or compete with the situated principles and values elaborated within the story being evaluated. Moreover, as Qvortrup and Nielsen (2019.:153) point out, while we 'dwell narratively, we rarely do so alone'. Like Qvortrup and Nielsen, who argue that the legitimacy and relevance of a given narrative is contingent on communal dwelling rather than reason and argument, Sadler (2022) maintains that narrative understandings are not first produced by individuals and then shared by communities; instead, they are always produced 'within an environment already structured by, and saturated with, other stories' (Sadler 2022:19). Stories are thus communal dwelling places. In inviting others to inhabit their stories, individual members of a community create the ground for identification and conscientia. In this sense, narrative rationality makes it possible for us to 'feel at home (dwell) in multiple stories' (Qvortrup and Nielsen 2019:159), allowing us to entertain various possibilities and narratives 'without being hindered by what constitutes a good argument' (Qvortrup and Nielsen 2019:160).

Applying this extended version of the narrative paradigm to medical decision making implies a need to incorporate a situated epistemological approach into EBM, one that recognizes and explains different types of rationality, and hence plural conceptualizations of evidence. It also calls for acknowledging the pre-reflective and practical nature of any experience of truth. This need not be seen in a negative light, for as Qvortrup and Nielsen explain, 'the experience of truth is tacit' and constitutes 'an opening that prompts engagement rather than a deterministic thought' (Qvortrup and Nielsen 2019:158). Finally, it suggests that we would do well to *know together* and *dwell together* by exchanging 'plots that are always in the process of re-creation rather than existing as settled scripts' (Fisher 1987:18). In the next section, we will look at how some of these extensions to the narrative paradigm might be conceptualized through the notion of narrative identification (McClure 2009).

6.3 Narrative Identification in the Age of Fragmented Narratives

In proposing the concept of *narrative identification*, McClure attempts to expand the narrative paradigm to better account for the fragmented, intertextual and syncretic character of personal and social narratives of identity, subjectivity and ideology, as emphasized by poststructuralist thinkers (McClure 2009:193). As we have seen, Fisher's narrative paradigm draws heavily on Kenneth Burke's notion of identification, treating it as the operative principle of narrative rationality (Fisher 1987:66). However, Fisher's intentions are undermined by the fact that the two concepts that are central to the narrative paradigm – probability and fidelity – are too dependent on 'normative notions of rationality' and too tied to the question of assessment 'to be fully descriptive of narrativity in general, especially in light of poststructuralism' (McClure 2009:193). By reducing identification to probability and fidelity, the narrative paradigm fails to account for how narratives interact, and how they may contain contradictory, unstable and implicit layers of meaning. As such, Fisher's use of the concept of identification is based on a paradox: on the one hand, he explicitly develops his theoretical alternative to the rational world paradigm by drawing on the notion of identification. On the other hand, he reintroduces the rational world paradigm by narrowing the process of identification to probability and fidelity (McClure 2009). Although Fisher includes in his definition of narration all 'symbolic actions – words and /or deeds – that have sequence and meaning for those who live, create and interpret them' (Fisher 1987:58), he also indirectly limits the concept to discourses that can measure up to the normative criteria of the rational world. As we saw earlier, Stroud argues that this limitation must be addressed in order for the narrative paradigm to accommodate and account for non-Western narratives such as those elaborated in ancient Indian didactic texts, which are multivalent in nature and do not persuade through the kind of consistency or coherence specified in Fisher's concept of narrative probablity (Stroud 2002:370). A similar argument can be made in terms of the narrative paradigm's failure to explain the more general discursive shift towards fragmented narratives as a prominent feature of postmodern consumption, both within and outside the West (Sadler 2022). Firat and Dholakia (1998), for instance, argue that fragmented televisual marketing communication deliberately lacks a coherent story and instead relies on the use of images that are only meant to 'leave the audience with a heightened sense of excitement about the product being marketed' (Firat and Dholakia 1998:80). Similarly, Sadler demonstrates how fragmented narratives on social media complicate the assessment of coherence. To assess the coherence of a fragment such as a single Twitter post in isolation is meaningless; the same fragment, moreover, may be understood by different audiences as part of both coherent and incoherent narrative wholes (Sadler 2022:137).

McClure argues that rather than being defined by appeal to the normative rationalities that underpin the concepts of probability and fidelity, we need to acknowledge that identification 'constitutes probability and fidelity'; that it is identification that 'makes possible the symbolic processes by which probability and fidelity are constituted" (McClure 2009:195; emphasis added). He thus distinguishes between Fisher's rationalistic understanding of identification and Burke's original definition; the latter implies that rationality itself is a rhetorical act that is dependent on the use of symbols to create meaning, and hence that 'all forms of rationality are composed via processes of identification' (McClure 2009:198). This approach to narrative identification is not normative: it is intended as a descriptive framework for assessing narratives critically to explain how they deploy symbolic processes of identification to appeal to audiences and secure their adherence (McClure 2009:201). McClure further insists that narrative identification is not achieved simply by engaging with a single narrative but involves mediation between several narratives in an intertextual exchange, recalling studies of intertextuality that demonstrate how 'multiple texts (narratives) intermingle in ways that are more akin to the processes of identification than traditional conceptions of narrative on which the narrative paradigm is constructed' (McClure 2009:199). Julia Kristeva's seminal work on intertextuality asserts that 'any text is constructed as a mosaic of quotations; any text is the absorption and transformation of another' (Kristeva 1980:66). A narrative therefore can never present a clear and stable meaning because it embodies societal conflicts and negotiations over meaning, in which utterances taken from various texts 'intersect with one another and neutralize one another' (Kristeva 1969:52; our translation). This suggests, too, that authors and receivers can never control the process of communication; they only contribute as mediators between recycled citations in an ongoing process of textual and intertextual productivity (Kristeva 1968). Narrative identification likewise evolves through a process of attending to an *internarrative productivity* rather than dwelling within a particular narrative.

McClure's critical analysis of Young Earth Creationism offers a good demonstration of this process. Despite substantial scientific evidence to the contrary, Young Earth Creationists maintain that the Earth is no more than 10,000 years old. McClure argues that it is not possible to account for widespread adherence to this narrative without taking into account a whole range of interrelated Biblical narratives as well as other religious and social narratives that intersect with them (McClure 2009:205–206). Because the unity of the text and the autonomy of the subject are illusions, McClure argues that fidelity is not necessarily produced by the narrative itself 'as if it was an isolatable attribute' of it. Instead, fidelity is to be understood as 'an act of constancy and personal attachment produced by agents to a *collection of narratives*'. Together these multiple narratives enable relations among members of an audience and produce 'texts and subjects in a sticky swirl that creates and sustains a community' (McClure 2009:207–208; emphasis added).

The Covid-19 controversies are similarly situated at the crossroads of multiple and conflicting stories. Rather than engaging in a detached, considered assessment of the coherence and fidelity of one specific narrative, we are continually negotiating our way through a multitude of narratives from a variety of medical and non-medical sources, often vascillating between conflicting accounts and reassessing their plausibility as we encounter new narratives. The purpose of the model of narrative analysis we have presented in this book is not to assist the reader in verifying a given story or stories. Instead, we hope that it will alert readers to the need to understand 'the strains that make alternative narratives inevitable' and encourage them to recognize 'the diversity of human frustrations, aspirations, satisfactions, and imaginative constructions' (Bennett and Edelman 1985:171).

6.4 A Final Note on Critical Appraisal in the EBM Model

To clarify the main argument we put forward in this book and guard against misunderstanding our claims, it is necessary to return briefly to the subject of critical appraisal in EBM. Burls (2009) offers a useful summary of the role of this process in EBM:

> When critically appraising research, it is important to first look for biases in the study; that is, whether the findings of the study might be due to the way the study was designed and carried out, rather than reflecting the truth.
>
> It is also important to remember that no study is perfect and free from bias; it is therefore necessary to systematically check that the researchers have done all they can to minimise bias.

Critical appraisal, as Burls' definition makes clear, is principally conceived as a methodological endeavour. It is intended as a tool for evaluating whether a given study is designed and conducted in a way that reduces (rather than fully eliminates) bias. Although Burls acknowledges that no study can totally escape bias, and hence no study can capture the absolute truth, the very idea of minimizing bias implies that there is an objective truth out there waiting to be discovered. The ontological presupposition that there is a world of hard facts that we can collect with varying degrees of success is not questioned. The whole idea of critical appraisal is therefore embedded within a rational world paradigm in which the world is conceived as a set of facts and logical puzzles that can be solved through appropriate analysis and the application of reason. We see the narrative paradigm as adding an ontological dimension to the concept of critical appraisal by casting the world as a set of stories that must be chosen among rather than facts to be discovered. In doing so, we do not set out to challenge the idea of appraising evidence from a methodological or epistemological perspective. Our claim is only that such appraisal is incomplete. The question 'What are the facts?' must be supplemented with another one: 'How do these facts make sense to people, and why?'. The latter is not about appraising the facts but about appraising the stories within which they are woven and acquire meaning.

Ultimately, we maintain, it is through narratives that knowledge about medical and other phenomena is communicated to others, enters the public space, and provokes discussion and disagreements. Importantly, effective narratives can enhance the reception of that knowledge and reduce some of the sources of resistance and misunderstanding that continue to plague public communication about important medical issues such as pandemics.

References

Abad-Santos, A. (2020) 'Performative masculinity is making American men sick', *Vox*, 10 August. Available at www.vox.com/platform/amp/the-goods/21356150/american-men-wont-wear-masks.

Agamben, G. (2020) 'Becoming faceless', *Autonomies*. Available at http://autonomies.org/2020/11/giorgio-agamben-becoming-faceless/.

Agamben, G. (2021) *Where Are We Now? The Epidemic as Politics*, translated by Valeria Dani, London: ERIS.

AHRQ (Agency for Healthcare Research and Quality) (2018) 2018 National Healthcare Quality and Disparities Report. Available at www.ahrq.gov/research/findings/nhqrdr/nhqdr18/index.html.

Alser, O., S. AlWaheidi, K. Elessi and H. Meghari (2020) 'COVID-19 in Gaza: a pandemic spreading in a place already under protracted lockdown', *Journal of East Mediterranean Health* 26(7): 762–763. DOI: https://doi.org/10.26719/emhj.20.089.

Alwan, N. A., R. A. Burgess, S. et al. (2020) 'Scientific consensus on the Covid-19 pandemic: we need to act now', *The Lancet* 396(10260): 71–72. DOI: https://doi.org/10.1016/S0140-6736(20)32153-X.

Andersen, H. (2012) 'Mechanisms: what are they evidence for in evidence-based medicine?', *Journal of Evaluation in Clinical Practice* 18 (5): 992–999.

Anguyo,I. and L. Storer (2020) 'In times of Covid-19 Kampala has become un-Ugandan', *LSE Blog*, 9 April. Available at https://blogs.lse.ac.uk/africaatlse/2020/04/09/kampala-epidemic-un-ugandan-society-in-times-covid-19/.

Anonymous (2021) 'ICU is full of the unvaccinated – my patience with them is wearing thin', *The Guardian*, 21 November. Available at www.theguardian.com/world/2021/nov/21/icu-is-full-of-the-unvaccinated-my-patience-with-them-is-wearing-thin.

Anslow, L. (2021) 'Lefties planted the anti-science seed fueling vaccine skepticism', *The Daily Beast*, 23 August. Available at www.thedailybeast.com/lefties-planted-the-anti-science-seed-fueling-vaccine-skepticism.

Anthony, A. (2020) 'Interview: Neil Ferguson: "I gave them an open goal to some extent"'. *The Guardian*, 6 December. Available at www.theguardian.com/world/2020/dec/06/professor-neil-ferguson-covid-modelling-epidemiologist-faces-of-2020.

Axe, D., W. M. Briggs and J. W. Richard (2020), *The Price of Panic: How the Tyranny of Experts Turned a Pandemic into a Catastrophe*, Regnery Publishing.

Bakan, J. (2003) *The Corporation: The Pathological Pursuit of Profit and Power*, Free Press.

Baker, M. (2006) *Translation and Conflict: A Narrative Account*, New York: Routledge.

Batt-Rawden, S. (2021) 'As a doctor, I think vaccines should be mandatory for healthcare workers', *Metro*, 3 April. Available at https://metro.co.uk/2021/04/03/as-a-doctor-i-would-support-mandatory-vaccines-for-healthcare-workers-14328670/.

Begum, T. (2020) Veiled racism: how the law change on Covid-19 face coverings makes Muslim women feel', *The Independent*, 26 June. Available at www.independent.co.uk/life-style/face-covering-mask-racism-muslim-hate-crime-niqab-burqa-a9587476.html.

Beioley, K., G. Parker, D. Strauss, A. Hancock and S. Venkataramakrishnan (2021) 'UK companies look to make Covid-19 vaccinations mandatory', *The Financial Times*, 16 February. Available at www.ft.com/content/965dfaf0-f070-4dae-93a6-28bedbdb75da.

Bellon, T. and E. M. Johnson (2021) 'From Boeing to Mercedes, a U.S. worker rebellion swells over vaccine mandates', *Reuters*, 2 November. Available at www.reuters.com/world/us/boeing-mercedes-us-worker-rebellion-swells-over-vaccine-mandates-2021-11-02/.

Bennett, W. L. and Edelman, M. (1985) 'Toward a new political narrative', *Journal of Communication* 35(4): 156–171.

Blunt, G. D. (2020) 'Face mask rules: do they really violate personal liberty?', *The Conversation*, 31 July. Available at https://the conversation.com/face-mask-rules-do-they-really-violate-personal-liberty-143634.

Bolsover, G. (2020) 'Balancing freedoms, rights and responsibilities during COVID in US: a study of anti- and pro-restriction discourse', *SSRN*, 4 August. DOI: http://dx .doi.org/10.2139/ssrn.3678626.

Brainard, J.S., N. Jones, I. Lake, L. Hooper and P. Hunter (2020) 'Facemasks and similar barriers to prevent respiratory illness such as COVID-19: a rapid systematic review'. *MedRxiv*. DOI: https://doi.org/10.1101/2020 .04.01.20049528.

Brewster, J. (2020) 'Trump again promotes experimental drug for coronavirus treatment hydroxychloroquine: "What do I know, I'm not a doctor. But I have common sense"', *Forbes Magazine*, 5 April. Available at www .forbes.com/sites/jackbrewster/2020/04/05/tr ump-again-promotes-experimental-drug-for -coronavirus-treatment-hydroxychloroquine-what-do-i-know-im-not-a-doctor-but-i-have-common-sense/? sh=5c53fe2f4609.

Broadbent, A. and B. T. H. Smart (2020) 'Why a one-size-fits-all approach to Covid-19 could have lethal consequences', *LSE Blog*, 27 March. Available at https://blogs.lse.ac.uk /africaatlse/2020/03/27/coronavirus-social-distancing-covid-19-lethal-consequences/.

Brookes, G. (2021) 'COVID-19 vaccines & genetic modification', *Open Access Government*, 3 June. Available at www .openaccessgovernment.org/covid-19-vaccines-genetic-modification/112020/.

Browne M (2018) 'Epistemic divides and ontological confusions', *Human Vaccines and Immunotherapeutics* 14(10): 2540–2542.

Bruner, J. (1991) 'The narrative construction of reality', *Critical Inquiry* 18(1): 1–21.

Bruton, M. (2020) *Morality, Epistemology, and Activism: How anti-vaccination advocates on Twitter construct a rhetoric of alternative immunity*, MA thesis, Indiana: Purdue University.

Burls, A. (2009) 'What is critical appraisal', *Evidence-Based Medicine*, second edition, Available at www.bandolier.org.uk/painres/do wnload/whatis/What_is_critical_appraisal.pdf.

Carothers, T. and B. Press (2020) 'The global rise of anti-lockdown protests – and what to do about it', *World Politics Review*. Available at www.worldpoliticsreview.com/articles/2913 7/amid-the-covid-19-pandemic-protest-movements-challenge-lockdowns-worldwide.

Carr, D. (2021) 'A virus without a world: the politics of science writing', *The Nation*, 7 September. Available at www .thenation.com/article/culture/carl-zimmer-virus/.

Cayley, D. (2020) 'The prognosis: looking the consequences in the eye', *Literary Review of Canada*, October. Available at https://review canada.ca/magazine/2020/10/the-prognosis/.

Chabal, E. (2021) 'The real reason France is skeptical of vaccines', *Foreign Policy*, 3 February. Available at https://foreignpolicy .com/2021/02/03/the-real-reason-france-is-skeptical-of-vaccines/.

Christiansen, A. T., M. M. Andersen and K. Kappel (2019) 'Are current EU policies on GMOs justified?', *Transgenic Research* 28: 267–286.

Clark, R. (2021) 'Austria will regret mandatory vaccinations', *The Spectator*, 19 November. Available at www.spectator.co.uk/article/aus tria-will-come-to-regret-mandatory-vaccinations.

Clarke, R. (2020) '"This man knows he's dying as surely as I do": a doctor's dispatches from the NHS frontline', *The Guardian*, 30 May. Available at www.theguardian.com/books/2 020/may/30/this-man-knows-hes-dying-as-surely-as-i-do-a-doctors-dispatches-from-intensive-care.

Collins, S. (2020) 'Trump's promotion of unproven drugs is cause for alarm, but not because he's making money off it', *Vox*, 7 April. Available at www.vox.com/2020/4/7/21211872 /trump-coronavirus-hydroxychloroquine-covid19-drugs-sanofi-owns.

Coman, J. (2020) 'Lockdown is breeding resentment. The right can see that – does the left?', *The Guardian*, 10 November. Available at www.theguardian.com/commentisfree/20 20/nov/10/populist-divisions-covid-nigel-farage-second-wave.

Cowburn, A. (2020) 'Neil Ferguson: Government coronavirus adviser quits after home visit from married lover', 5 May. Available at www .independent.co.uk/news/uk/politics/neil-ferguson-resigns-coronavirus-antonia-staats-social-distancing-government-a9500581.html.

Cullen, P. (2021) 'GP suspended by Medical Council over refusal to give Covid-19 vaccine', *The Irish Times*, 22 March. Available at www.irishtimes.com/news/heal th/gp-suspended-by-medical-council-over-refusal-to-give-covid-19-vaccine-1 .4516239.

Czypionka, T., T. Greenhalgh, D. Bassler and M. B. Bryant (2020) 'Masks and face coverings for the lay public: a narrative update', *Annals of Internal Medicine*. DOI: h ttps://doi.org/10.7326/M20-6625.

Dangor, Z. and F. Sucker (2021) 'South Africa has the legal tools to challenge the vaccine nationalism of rich countries', *Daily Maverick*, 25 January. Available at www .dailymaverick.co.za/article/2021-01-25-south-africa-has-the-legal-tools-to-challenge -the-vaccine-nationalism-of-rich-countries/.

Dawber, A. (2013) 'Israel gave birth control to Ethiopian Jews without their consent', *The Independent*, 27 January. Available at www .independent.co.uk/news/world/middle-east /israel-gave-birth-control-to-ethiopian-jews-without-their-consent-8468800.html.

Deer, B. (2020) *The Doctor Who Fooled the World: Andrew Wakefield's War on Vaccines*, London: Scribe Publications.

Deoni, S. C. L., J. Beauchemin, A. Volpe and V. D'Sa (2021) 'Impact of the COVID-19 pandemic on early child cognitive development: initial findings in a longitudinal observational study of child health', *medRxiv*. DOI: https://doi.org/10 .1101/2021.08.10.21261846.

Department of Education (2021) 'Face coverings in education'. Available at https://assets .publishing.service.gov.uk/government/upload s/system/uploads/attachment_data/file/967285 /Face_coverings_in_education-March-2021 .pdf.

Devlin, K. (2020) 'Boris Johnson calls face masks in schools "nonsensical" hours after latest U-turn', *The Independent*, 26 August. Available at www.independent.co.uk/news/u k/politics/boris-johnson-face-masks-school-classroom-children-covid-19-a9689741.html.

Dominus, S. (2020) 'The Covid drug wars that pitted doctor vs doctor', *The New York Times*, 5 August. Available at www.nytimes.com/20 20/08/05/magazine/covid-drug-wars-doctors.html.

Eaton, L. (2021) 'Covid-19: WHO warns against "vaccine nationalism" or face further virus mutations', *BMJ* 373:n292. Available at www .bmj.com/content/372/bmj.n292.

Ekeløve-Slydal, G. and L. H. Kvanvig (2020) 'Lockdowns vs. religious freedom: COVID-19 is a trust building exercise', OpenGlobalRights. Available at www .openglobalrights.org/lockdowns-vs-religious-freedom-covid-19-is-a-trust-building-exercise/.

Elgot, J. and J. Halliday (2020) 'Boris Johnson drops advice against face mask use in English schools', *The Guardian*, 25 August. Available at www.theguardian.com/world/2020/aug/2 5/boris-johnson-drops-advice-against-face-mask-use-in-english-schools.

Elmer, S. (2020) 'The science and law of refusing to wear masks: texts and arguments in support of civil disobedience', *Architects for Social Housing*, 11 June. Available at https:// architectsforsocialhousing.co.uk/2020/06/11 /the-science-and-law-of-refusing-to-wear-masks-texts-and-arguments-in-support-of-civil-disobedience/.

Engebretsen, E. and O. P. Ottersen (2021) 'Vaccine inequities, intellectual property rights and pathologies of power in the global response to COVID-19', *International Journal of Health Policy Management*. DOI: 10.34172/ijhpm.2021.57.

Engebretsen, E., K. Heggen, S. Wieringa and T. Greenhalgh (2016) 'Uncertainty and objectivity in clinical decision making: a clinical case in emergency medicine', *Medicine, Health Care and Philosophy* 19(4): 595–603.

Engebretsen, E., N. Køpke Vøllestad, A. Klopstad Wahl, S. Robinson and K. Heggen (2015) 'Unpacking the process of interpretation in evidence-based decision making', *Journal of Evaluation in Clinical Practice* 21(3): 529.

Euronews (2021) 'COVID-19: Austria begins nationwide lockdown for unvaccinated people', 15 November. Available at www .euronews.com/2021/11/14/covid-19-austrian-government-orders-lockdown-for-unvaccinated.

Evans, D. (2003) 'Hierarchy of evidence: a framework for ranking evidence evaluating healthcare interventions', *Journal of Clinical Nursing* 12(1): 77–84.

Fancourt, D., A. Steptoe and L. Wright (2020) 'The Cummings effect: politics, trust, and behaviours during the COVID-19 pandemic', *The Lancet* 396(10249): 464–465.

Felix, G. (2020) 'Wearing a face mask helps protect me against Covid-19, but not against racism', *STAT*, 13 May. Available at www.statnews.com/2020/05/13/black-man-think-twice-wearing-face-mask-in-public-racism/.

Feng, E. and A. Cheng (2020) 'Restrictions and rewards: how China is locking down half a billion citizens', *NPR*, 21 February. Available at www.npr.org/sections/goatsandsoda/2020/02/21/806958341/restrictions-and-rewards-how-china-is-locking-down-half-a-billion-citizens?t=1621332600454.

Firat, A. F. and N. Dholakia (1998) *Consuming People: From Political Economy to Matters of Consumption*, New York: Routledge.

Fisher, W. R. (1984) 'Narration as a human communication paradigm: the case of public moral agreement', *Communication Monographs* 51: 1–22.

Fisher, W. R. (1985a) 'The narrative paradigm: an elaboration', *Communication Monographs* 52: 347–367.

Fisher, W. R. (1985b) 'The narrative paradigm: in the beginning', *Journal of Communication* 35(4): 74–89.

Fisher, W. R. (1987) *Human Communication as Narration: Toward a Philosophy of Reason, Value, and Action*, Columbia, South Carolina: University of South Carolina Press.

Fisher, W. R. (1994) 'Narrative rationality and the logic of scientific discourse', *Argumentation* 8: 21–32.

Fisher, W. R. (1995) 'Narration, knowledge, and the possibility of wisdom', in W. R. Fisher and R. F. Goodman (eds.) *Rethinking Knowledge: Reflections across the Disciplines*, New York: State University of New York Press, 169–192.

Fisher, W. R. (1997) 'Narration, reason, and community', in L. P. Hinchman and S. K. Hinchman (eds.) *Memory, Identity, Community: The Idea of Narrative in the Human Sciences*, Albany: State University of New York Press, 307–327.

Forman, R., S. Shah, P. Jeurissen, M. Jit and E. Mossialos (2021) 'COVID-19 vaccine challenges: what have we learned so far and what remains to be done?', *Health Policy* 125 (5): 553–567.

Frank, A. (1995) *The Wounded Storyteller: Body, Illness and Ethics*, Chicago: University of Chicago Press.

Franklin County Public Health (2020) 'COVID-19 general guidance on wearing face mask for African Americans and communities of color, April'. Available at https://vax2normal.org/wp-content/uploads/2020/05/Face_Mask_Racial_Equity_April.pdf.

Gandhi, M. (2016) *A Guide to Health*, New Delhi: Ocean Books.

Gaskin, I. M. (2003) *Ina May's Guide to Childbirth*. New York: Bantam.

Goodman, B. (2020) 'The forgotten science behind face masks', *WebMD*. Available at www.webmd.com/lung/news/20200826/the-forgotten-science-behind-face-masks.

Greenhalgh, T. (2016) *Cultural Contexts of Health: The Use of Narrative Research in the Health Sector*, Copenhagen: WHO Regional Office for Europe; (Health Evidence Network (HEN) synthesis report 49).

Greenhalgh, T. (2020a) 'Face coverings for the lay public: an alternative view', The Centre for Evidence-Based Medicine, 27 May. Available at www.cebm.net/covid-19/face-coverings-for-the-lay-public-an-alternative-view/.

Greenhalgh, T. (2020b) 'Face coverings for the public: laying straw men to rest', *Journal of Evaluation in Clinical Practice* 26(4): 1070–1077.

Greenhalgh, T. and J. Howard (2020) 'Masks for all? The science says yes'. *fast.ai*. Available at www.fast.ai/2020/04/13/masks-summary/.

Greenhalgh, T., J. Howick and N. Maskrey N (2014) 'Evidence based medicine: a movement in crisis?', *BMJ* 348: g3725. DOI: https://doi.org/10.1136/bmj.g3725.

Greenhalgh, T., M. McKee and M. Kelly-Irving (2020) 'Opinion: the pursuit of herd immunity is a folly: so who's funding this bad science?', *The Guardian*, 18 October. Available at www.theguardian.com/commentisfree/2020/oct/18/covid-herd-immunity-funding-bad-science-anti-lockdown.

Gust, D., C. Brown, K. Sheedy, et al. (2005) 'Immunization attitudes and beliefs among parents: beyond a dichotomous perspective', *American Journal of Health Behavior* 29: 81–92.

Hacking I. (2001) *An Introduction to Probability and Inductive Logic*, Cambridge: Cambridge University Press.

Harsin, J. (2020) 'Toxic white masculinity, post-truth politics and the Covid-19 infodemic', *European Journal of Cultural Studies* 23(6): 1060–1068.

Hasan, M. (2020) 'The coronavirus is empowering islamophobes: but exposing the idiocy of islamophobia', *The Intercept*, 14 April. Available at https://theintercept.com/2020/04/14/coronavirus-muslims-islamophobia/.

Hawker, L. (2021) 'Captain Tom Moore's Barbados holiday: how trip completed a life-long dream for NHS hero', *Express*, 3 February. Available at www.express.co.uk/news/uk/1392458/tom-moore-barbados-holiday-trip-captain-tom-moore-dead-latest.

Hedgecoe, G. (2020) 'Coronavirus: Spain's children run free from lockdown – but not all', *BBC News*, 26 April. Available at www.bbc.com/news/world-europe-52409407.

Heidegger, M. (2010) *Being and Time*, translated by Joan Stambaugh, Albany, NY: State University of New York Press.

Hendrix, S. and S. Rubin (2021) 'Violence erupts in Israel's ultra-Orthodox neighborhoods over coronavirus restrictions', *The Washington Post*, 26 January. Available at www.washingtonpost.com/world/middle_east/ultra-orthodox-israel-police-covid/2021/01/25/2438e840-5ee3-11eb-a177-7765f29a9524_story.html.

Henry, E. (2021) 'All businesses are essential', *EIN Presswire*, 11 January. Available at www.einpresswire.com/article/534346395/all-businesses-are-essential.

Hickman, T. (2020) 'The use and misuse of guidance during the UK's Coronavirus lockdown', 4 September, SSRN. Available at https://papers.ssrn.com/sol3/papers.cfm?abstract_id=3686857.

Hitchins, P. (2020) 'Face masks turn us into voiceless submissives – and it's not science forcing us to wear them, it's politics', *The Daily Mail*, 19 July. Available at www.dailymail.co.uk/debate/article-8537489/PETER-HITCHENS-Face-masks-turn-voiceless-submissives.html.

Hollihan, T. and P. Riley (1987) 'The rhetorical power of a compelling story: a critique of a 'toughlove' parental support group', *Communication Quarterly* 35(1): 13–25.

Homer, R. (2021) 'Covax misses its 2021 delivery target – what's gone wrong in the fight against vaccine nationalism?', *The Conversation*, 17 September. Available at https://theconversation.com/covax-misses-its-2021-delivery-target-whats-gone-wrong-in-the-fight-against-vaccine-nationalism-167753?utm_medium=email&utm_campaign=Latest%20from%20The%20Conversation%20for%20September%202020%202021%20-%202064720367&utm_content=Latest%20from%20The%20Conversation%20for%20September%202020%202021%20-%2020264720367+CID_7733bf2baea34866c054eb b44819073c&utm_source=campaign_monitor_uk&utm_term=Covax%20misses%20its%202021%20delivery%20target%20%20whats%20gone%20wrong%20in%20the%20fight%20against%20vaccine%20nationalism.

Jamison, A. M., S. C. Quinn and V. S. Freimuth (2019) '"You don't trust a government vaccine": narratives of institutional trust and influenza vaccination among African American and white adults', *Social Science & Medicine* 221: 87–94.

Jiang, S. (2020) 'Don't rush to deploy COVID-19 vaccines and drugs without sufficient safety guarantees', *Nature* 579: 321.

Kaebnick, G. E. and M. Gusmano (2019) 'Forget about "because science"', *Slate*, 15 April. Available at https://slate.com/technology/2019/04/vaccination-values-science-based-policy.html.

Kagumire, J. R. (2021) 'The colonial overtones of omicron travel bans', *Al Jazeera*, 6 December. Available at www.aljazeera.com/opinions/2021/12/6/the-colonial-roots-of-western-responses-to-omicron.

Kahn, J. P., L. M. Henry, A. C. Mastroianni, W. H. Chen and R. Macklin (2020) 'For now, it's unethical to use human challenge studies for SARS-CoV-2 vaccine development', *Proceedings of the National Academy of Sciences of the United States of America* 117 (46): 28538–28542. DOI: https://doi.org/10.1073/pnas.2021189117.

Keene, D. R. (2020) 'Does the lockdown breach the right to freedom of religion?', *UK Human Rights Blog*, 30 November. Available at https://ukhumanrightsblog.com/2020/11/30/does-the-lockdown-breach-the-right-to-freedom-of-religion/.

Kennedy, J. (2019) 'Populist politics and vaccine hesitancy in Western Europe', *European Journal of Public Health* 29(3): 512–516.

Khan, A. (2021) 'What is 'vaccine nationalism' and why is it so harmful?', *Aljazeera*, 7 February. Available at www.aljazeera.com/features/2021/2/7/what-is-vaccine-nationalism-and-why-is-it-so-harmful.

Kim, T. (2018) 'Goldman Sachs asks in biotech research report: "Is curing patients a sustainable business model?"', *CNBC*, 11 April. Available at www.cnbc.com/2018/04/11/goldman-asks-is-curing-patients-a-sustainable-business-model.html.

Kirkwood, W. G. (1992) 'Narrative and the rhetoric of possibility', *Communication Monographs* 59(1): 30–47.

Kristeva, J. (1968) 'La productivité dite texte', *Communications* 11(1): 59–83.

Kristeva, J. (1969) *Semeiotiké: recherches pour une sémanalyse*, Paris: Points.

Kristeva, J. (1980) *Desire in Language: A Semiotic Approach to Literature and Art*, New York: Columbia University Press.

Kristian, B. (2020) 'The strange conflation of masks and masculinity', *The Week*, 14 May. Available at https://theweek.com/articles/914223/strange-conflation-masks-masculinity.

Kum, D. (2020) 'Fueled by a history of mistreatment, Black Americans distrust the new COVID-19 vaccines', *Time*, 28 December. Available at https://time.com/5925074/black-americans-covid-19-vaccine-distrust/.

Lagman, J. D. N. (2021) 'Vaccine nationalism: a predicament in ending the COVID-19 pandemic', *Journal of Public Health* 43(2): e375–e376. DOI: https://doi.org/10.1093/pubmed/fdab088.

Larson, H. J. (2020) *Stuck: How Vaccine Rumors Start – and Why They Don't Go Away*, Oxford: Oxford University Press.

Lazarus, J. V., S. C. Ratzan, A. Palayew *et al.* (2021) 'A global survey of potential acceptance of a COVID-19 vaccine', *Nature Medicine* 27: 225–228.

Lee, T. and C. Holt (2021) 'Intellectual property, COVID-19 vaccines, and the proposed TRIPS waiver', *American Action Forum*, 10 May. Available at www.americanactionforum.org/insight/intellectual-property-covid-19-vaccines-and-the-proposed-trips-waiver/#ixzz770IqwWVm.

Lewis, N. (2020) 'The dangerous rise of rule by experts', *Spiked*, 28 April. Available at www.spiked-online.com/2020/04/28/the-dangerous-rise-of-rule-by-experts/.

Linnane, C. (2021) 'Austria locks down its unvaccinated, and Netherlands reimposes restrictions, as Europe battles surge in COVID cases', *MarketWatch*, 15 November. Available at www.marketwatch.com/story/austria-locks-down-its-unvaccinated-and-netherlands-reimposes-restrictions-as-europe-battles-surge-in-covid-cases-11636990781.

Lonergan, B. (1992) *Insight. A Study of Human Understanding*, Toronto: University of Toronto Press.

Lowe, Y. (2020) 'Gang members wearing coronavirus medical masks to disguise themselves', *The Telegraph*, 21 March. Available at www.telegraph.co.uk/news/2020/03/21/gang-members-wearing-coronavirus-medical-masks-disguise/.

Mallapaty, S. (2021) 'Omicron-variant border bans ignore the evidence, say scientists', *Nature*, 2 December. Available at www.nature.com/articles/d41586-021-03608-x.

Malone, K. M. and A. R. Hinman (2007) 'Vaccination mandates: the public health imperative and individual rights', in R. A. Goodman, R. E. Hoffman, W. Lopez et al. (eds.) *Law in Public Health Practice*, Oxford: Oxford University Press. Available at www.cdc.gov/vaccines/imz-managers/guides-pubs/downloads/vacc_mandates_chptr13.pdf.

Marcus, J. (2020) 'The dudes who won't wear masks', *The Atlantic*, 23 June. Available at www.theatlantic.com/ideas/archive/2020/06/dudes-who-wont-wear-masks/613375/.

Martin, G., E. Hanna and R. Dingwall (2020a) 'Response to Greenhalgh et al.: face masks, the precautionary principle, and evidence-informed policy', *BMJ* 369: m1435. DOI: https://doi.org/10.1136/bmj.m1435.

Mayta, R., K. K. Shailaja and A. Nyong'o (2021) 'Vaccine nationalism is killing us. We need an internationalist approach', *The Guardian*, 17 June. Available at www.theguardian.com/commentisfree/2021/jun/17/covid-vaccine-nationalism-internationalist-approach.

McBee, T. P. (2019) 'Toxic masculinity is under attack. That's fine', *Vox*, 22 January. Available at www.vox.com/first-person/2019/1/22/1818

8776/toxic-masculinity-gillette-ad-apa-guidelines.

McClure, K. (2009) 'Resurrecting the narrative paradigm: identification and the case of Young Earth Creationism', *Rhetoric Society Quarterly* 39(2): 189–211.

McGee, M. C. and J. S. Nelson (1985) 'Narrative reason in public argument', *Journal of Communication* 35(4): 139–155.

McKelvey, T. (2020) 'Coronavirus: why are Americans so angry about masks?', *BBC News*, 20 July. Available at www.bbc.com/news/world-us-canada-53477121.

Merleau-Ponty, M. (1962) *Phenomenology of Perception*, translated from the French by Colin Smith, New York: Routledge.

Mezzadra, S. and M. Stierl (2020) 'What happens to freedom of movement during a pandemic?', *OpenDemocracy*, 24 March. Available at www.opendemocracy.net/en/can-europe-make-it/what-happens-freedom-movement-during-pandemic/.

Milko, V. (2020) 'Concern among Muslims over halal status of COVID-19 vaccine', *ABC News*, 20 December. Available at https://abcnews.go.com/Health/wireStory/concern-muslims-halal-status-covid-19-vaccine-74826269.

Morgan, W. (2021) 'Anti-vaxxers are weaponising the vaccine hesitancy of Black communities', *The Conversation*, 26 January. Available at https://tinyurl.com/nrka2vca.

Morooka, J. (2002) 'Bourdieusean criticism of the narrative paradigm: the case of historical texts', *ISSA Porceedings 2002*. Available at https://rozenbergquarterly.com/issa-proceedings-2002-bourdieuian-criticism-of-the-narrative-paradigm-the-case-of-historical-textsi/?print=pdf.

Muller, J. Z. (2018) *The Tyranny of Metrics*. Princeton, NJ: Princeton University Press.

Munroe, S. (2020) 'Commentary: with liberty and face masks for all', *The Herald*, 16 August. Available at www.heraldnet.com/opinion/commentary-with-liberty-and-face-masks-for-all/.

Murphy, R. (2020) 'The Great Barrington Declaration has nothing to do with epidemiology and a great deal to do with far right economics', *Brave New Europe*, 13 October. Available at https://braveneweurope.com/richard-murphy-the-great-barrington-declaration-has-nothing-to-do-with-epidemiology-and-a-great-deal-to-do-with-far-right-economics.

NIPH (2020a) 'Recommendations about face masks', 14 August. Available at www.fhi.no/en/archive/covid-19-archive/COVID-19-archived-news-from-2020/aug/recommendations-about-face-masks/.

NIPH (2020b) 'Face masks and visor use by the general public', 29 October. Available at www.fhi.no/en/op/novel-coronavirus-facts-advice/facts-and-general-advice/munnbind-i-befolkningen/.

O'Brien, K. (2020) 'Are coronavirus policies aiding criminal activity', *Colligan Law*, 3 June. Available at https://insights.colliganlaw.com/post/102g8o2/are-coronavirus-policies-aiding-criminal-activity.

O'Connor, R. (2021) '"Conscientious objector" Irish GP suspended by Medical Council for refusing to vaccinate patients', *The Irish Post*, 22 March. Available at www.irishpost.com/news/conscientious-objector-irish-gp-suspended-by-medical-council-for-refusing-to-vaccinate-patients-207027.

O'Grady, S. (2021) 'This is what we do about anti-vaxxers: No job. No entry. No NHS access', *The Independent*, 18 May. Available at www.independent.co.uk/voices/antivaxxers-vaccine-coronavirus-nhs-b1849437.html.

Olmstead, M. (2021) 'Why a prominent group of Catholic bishops is objecting to the Johnson & Johnson vaccine', *Slate*, 4 March. Available at https://slate.com/human-interest/2021/03/johnson-and-johnson-vaccine-catholic-bishops-objections.html.

Omer, S. B. (2020) 'The discredited doctor hailed by the anti-vaccine movement', *Nature*, 27 October. Doi: https://doi.org/10.1038/d41586-020-02989-9.

Orange, R. (2020) 'As the rest of Europe lives under lockdown, Sweden keeps calm and carries on', *The Guardian*, 28 March. Available at www.theguardian.com/world/2020/mar/28/as-the-rest-of-europe-lives-under-lockdown-sweden-keeps-calm-and-carries-on.

Pabst, A. (2021) 'Rethinking evidence-based policy', *National Institute Economic Review* 255: 85–91.

Philipose, R. (2020) 'Covid-19: a look at anti-mask rallies held around the world amid the pandemic', *The Indian Express*, 6 September.

Available at https://indianexpress.com/art icle/world/covid-19-a-look-at-anti-mask-rallies-held-around-the-world-amid-the-pandemic-6585722/.

Phillips, T. (2020) 'Brazil: Bolsonaro reportedly uses homophobic slur to mock masks', *The Guardian*, 8 July. Available at www .theguardian.com/world/2020/jul/08/bolso naro-masks-slur-brazil-coronavirus.

PopMatters (2020) '"Anti-vaxxers: how to challenge a misinformed movement": excerpt', 9 September. Available at www .popmatters.com/jonathan-m-berman-anti-vaxxers-2647525642.html? rebelltitem=1#rebelltitem1.

Press Association (2021) 'Boris Johnson says sorry for not wearing mask on hospital visit', *The Free Press*, 17 November. Available at www.denbighshirefreepress.co.uk/news/nat ional/19723707.boris-johnson-says-sorry-not-wearing-mask-hospital-visit/.

Qvortrup, M. and E. B. Nielsen (2019) 'Dwelling narratively: exploring Heideggerian perspectives in the narrative paradigm', *Philosophy and Rhetoric* 52(2): 142–162.

Repucci, S. and A. Slipowitz (2020) 'Democracy under lockdown', Freedom House. Available at https://freedomhouse.org/report/special-report/2020/democracy-under-lockdown.

Richards, J. W., D. Axe and W. M. Briggs (2020) 'Covid-19: the tyranny of experts', *Religion & Liberty* 30(4), 23 October. Available at https:// www.acton.org/religion-liberty/volume-30-number-4/covid-19-tyranny-experts.

Roberts, K.G. (2004) 'Texturing the narrative paradigm: folklore and communication', *Communication Quarterly* 52(2): 129–142.

Rone, J. (2021) 'Social media disinformation and vaccine hesitancy: it's more complicated than that', *power-switch*, blog of the Minderoo Centre for Technology and Democracy, University of Cambridge, 13 February. Available at https://powerswitchorg .wordpress.com/2021/02/13/social-media-disinformation-and-vaccine-hesitancy-its-more-complicated-than-that/.

Rowland, R. (1987) 'Narrative: mode of discourse or paradigm', *Communication Monographs* 54: 264–275.

Rutschman, A. S. (2020) 'The reemergence of vaccine nationalism', *Georgetown Journal of International Affairs*, 3 July. Available at https://gjia.georgetown.edu/2020/07/03/the-reemergence-of-vaccine-nationalism/.

Rutter, H., M. Wolpert and T. Greenhalgh (2020) 'Managing uncertainty in the Covid-19 era', *BMJ* 370: m3349. DOI: https:// doi.org/10.1136/bmj.m3349.

Sackett, D. L., M. C. W. Rosenberg, M. Gray, B. R. Haynes and S. W. Richardson (1996) 'Evidence based medicine: what it is and what it isn't', *BMJ* 312(7023): 71–72.

Sadler, N. (2022) *Fragmented Narrative; Telling and Interpreting Stories in the Twitter Age*, New York: Routledge.

Sample, I. (2021) 'Vaccine hesitancy in some health workers in England "may undermine rollout"', *The Guardian*, 14 February. Available at www.theguardian.com/world/2 021/feb/14/vaccine-rollout-caution-some-health-workers-england.

Schofield, K. (2020) 'Coronavirus: wearing face masks makes no difference to spread of disease, insists UK medical chief', *PoliticsHome*, 3 April. Available at www .politicshome.com/news/article/corona virus-wearing-face-masks-makes-no-difference-to-spread-of-disease-insists-uk-medical-chief.

Schurman, R. and W. Munro (2009) 'Targeting capital: a cultural economy approach to understanding the efficacy of two anti-genetic engineering movements', *AJS: American Journal of Sociology* 115(1): 155–202.

Schwab, T. (2020) 'Are Bill Gates's billions distorting public health data?', *The Nation*, 3 December. Available at www .thenation.com/article/society/gates-covid-data-ihme/.

Shell, E. R. (2020) 'Act now, wait for perfect evidence later, says 'high priestess' of UK. Covid-19 masking campaign', *Science*. Available at www-sciencemag-org.ezproxy.uio.no/news/2020/10/act-now-wait-perfect-evidence-later-says-high-priestess -uk-covid-19-masking-campaign.

Shields, B. (2021) 'AstraZeneca creator says Australia's mixed messages on vaccine may cost lives', *The Sydney Morning Herald*, 30 July. Available at www.smh.com.au/worl d/europe/astrazeneca-creator-says-australia-s-mixed-messages-on-vaccine-may-cost-lives-20210730-p58e8v.html.

Siddiqui, Z. (2021) 'In Pakistan, legacy of fake CIA vaccination programs leads to vaccine hesitancy', *Vice* (World News), 9 March. Available at www.vice.com/amp/en/article/5 dpvkd/in-pakistan-legacy-of-fake-cia-vaccination-programs-leads-to-vaccine-hesitancy?__twitter_impression=true.

Siegel, E. (2017) 'The real problem with Charles Murray and "The Bell Curve"', *Scientific American*, 12 April. Available at https://blogs.scientificamerican.com/voices/the-real-problem-with-charles-murray-and-the-bell-curve/.

Sky News (2021) 'Microsoft founder Bill Gates warns of bioterrorist attacks and urges world leaders to use "germ games" to prepare in interview with Jeremy Hunt', 6 November. Available at https://news.sky.com/story/microsoft-founder-bill-gates-warns-of-bioterrorist-attacks-and-urges-world-leaders-to-use-germ-games-to-prepare-in-interview-with-jeremy-hunt-12459391.

Smith, C. (2021) 'Plagues and classical history – what the humanities will tell us about COVID in years to come', *The Conversation*, 11 August. Available at https://theconversation.com/plagues-and-classical-history-what-the-humanities-will-tell-us-about-covid-in-years-to-come-165848?utm_medium=email&utm_campaign=Latest%20from%20The%20Conversation%20for%20August%2012%202021%20-%202029219951&utm_content=Latest%20from%20The%20Conversation%20for%20August%2012%202021%20-%202029219951+CID_f7780761e36e4c1708b6ec4dee6c7f6a&utm_source=campaign_monitor_uk&utm_term=how%20history%20tends%20to%20play%20out.

Snowdon, C. J. (2021) 'Rise of the coronavirus cranks'. *Quillette*, 16 January. Available at https://quillette.com/2021/01/16/rise-of-the-coronavirus-cranks/.

Solomon, M. (2015) *Making Medical Knowledge*, Oxford: Oxford University Press.

Soucheray, S. (2020) 'Controversy on Covid-19 mask study spotlights messiness of science during a pandemic', CIDRAP (Centre for Infectious Disease Research and Policy), 24 June. Available at www.cidrap.umn.edu/news-perspective/2020/06/controversy-covid-19-mask-study-spotlights-messiness-science-during.

Spitzer, M. (2020) 'Masked education? The benefits and burdens of wearing face masks in schools during the current Corona pandemic', *Trends in Neuroscience and Education* 20: 100138 . DOI: https://10.1016/j.tine.2020.100138.

Sridhar, G. (2020) 'Continual lockdowns are not the answer to bringing covid under control', *The Guardian*, 10 October. Available at https://amp.theguardian.com/commentisfree/2020/oct/10/continual-local-lockdowns-answer-covid-control?__twitter_impression=true.

Stache, L. C. (2018) 'Fisher narrative paradigm', in M. Allen (ed.) *The SAGE Encyclopedia of Communication Research Methods*, Thousand Oaks: Sage, 576–578.

Stengers, I. (2013) *Sciences et pouvoirs: la démocratie face à la technoscience*. La Découverte.

Stevenson, A. (2021) '"My body is a temple": vaccine hesitancy, religious exemptions, and the integrity of Christian witness', *ABC*, 11 October. Available at www.abc.net.au/religion/vaccines-religious-exemptions-and-christian-witness/13580026.

Stewart, H. (2020) 'Neil Ferguson: UK coronavirus adviser resigns after breaking lockdown rules', *The Guardian*, 5 May. Available at www.theguardian.com/uk-news/2020/may/05/uk-coronavirus-adviser-prof-neil-ferguson-resigns-after-breaking-lockdown-rules.

Storer, L. and K. Dawson (2020) 'Perspectives from Uganda's borders on containing COVID-19', *LSE Blog*, 8 April. Available at https://blogs.lse.ac.uk/africaatlse/2020/04/08/perspectives-from-ugandas-borders-on-containing-covid-19/.

Strong, G. (2021) 'Captain Sir Tom Moore's family are "hurt" by cruel Barbados comments', *Hello*, 3 February. Available at www.hellomagazine.com/celebrities/20210203106000/captain-sir-tom-moore-family-hurt-barbados-comments/.

Stroud, S. R. (2002) 'Multivalent narratives: extending the narrative paradigm with insights from ancient Indian philosophical texts', *Western Journal of Communication* 66 (3): 369–393.

Stroud, S. R. (2016) 'Narrative rationality', in K. B. Jensen and R. T. Craig (eds.) *The International Encyclopedia of Communication Theory and Philosophy*, John Wiley. DOI: 10.1002/9781118766804.wbiect050.

Susam-Sarajeva, Ş. (2020) 'Translating birth stories as counter narratives', *Mutatis Mutandis* 13(1): 45–63.

Talic, S., S. Shah, H. Wild et al. (2021) 'Effectiveness of public health measures in reducing the incidence of covid-19, SARS-CoV-2 transmission, and covid-19 mortality', *BMJ* 375: e068302. DOI: https://doi-org.ezproxy.uio.no/10.1136/bmj-2021-068302.

Tang, J. (2020) 'Expert reaction to Barrington Declaration, an open letter arguing against lockdown policies and for 'Focused Protection'', *Science Media Centre*, 6 October. Available at www.sciencemediacentre.org/expert-reaction-to-barrington-declaration-an-open-letter-arguing-against-lockdown-policies-and-for-focused-protection/.

Tavernise, S. (2021) 'Vaccine skepticism was viewed as a knowledge problem. It's actually about gut beliefs', *The New York Times*, 6 May. Available at www.nytimes.com/2021/04/29/us/vaccine-skepticism-beliefs.html.

Theobald, B. (2019) 'A 1970 law led to the mass sterilization of native American women. That history still matters', *Time*, 28 November. Available at https://time.com/5737080/native-american-sterilization-history/.

Tilley, H. (2020) 'COVID-19 across Africa: colonial hangovers, racial hierarchies, and medical histories', *Journal of West African History* 6(2): 155–179.

Timmermans, S. and M. Berg (2003) *The Gold Standard: The Challenge of Evidence-Based Medicine and Standardization in Health Care*, Philadelphia: Temple University Press.

Torjesen, I. (2020) 'Covid-19: pre-purchasing vaccine – sensible or selfish?', *BMJ* 370: m3226. DOI: https://doi.org/10.1136/bmj.m3226.

Urrutia, M. L. (2021) 'COVID data is complex and changeable – expecting the public to heed it as restrictions ease is optimistic', *The Conversation*, 16 July. Available at https://theconversation.com/covid-data-is-complex-and-changeable-expecting-the-public-to-heed-it-as-restrictions-ease-is-optimistic-164609?utm_medium=email&utm_campaign=Latest%20from%20The%20Conversation%20for%20July%2019%202021%20-%202006519710&utm_content=Latest%20from%20The%20Conversation%20for%20July%2019%2021%20-%202006519710+CID_31cb25906c f5587437ba1e4758e56645&utm_source=campaign_monitor_uk&utm_term=make%20sense%20of%20all%20the%20data.

Veneza, R. (2021) ''I find it puzzling': Religious involvement in anti-lockdown protests at odds with other congregations', *CTV News*, 11 May. Available at https://kitchener.ctvnews.ca/i-find-it-puzzling-religious-involvement-in-anti-lockdown-protests-at-odds-with-other-congregations-1.5423862.

Vogel, G. (2020) 'It's been so, so surreal.' Critics of Sweden's lax pandemic policies face fierce backlash', *Science*, 6 October. Available at www.science.org/content/article/it-s-been-so-so-surreal-critics-sweden-s-lax-pandemic-policies-face-fierce-backlash.

Walker, A. (2020) 'National talk radio hosts reject calls for masks, echoed by local hosts in at least one coronavirus hot spot', *Mediamatters for America*, 7 February. Available at www.mediamatters.org/coronavirus-covid-19/national-talk-radio-hosts-reject-calls-masks-echoed-local-hosts-least-one.

Walravens, T. and P. O'Shea (2021) 'Covid: Why are Swedish towns banning masks?', *The Conversation*, 8 February. Available at www.news24.com/health24/medical/infectious-diseases/coronavirus/covid-why-are-swedish-towns-banning-masks-20210211.

Warnick, B. (1987) 'The narrative paradigm: another story', *Quarterly Journal of Speech* 73: 172–182.

Weiner, S., K. Lavery and D. Nardi (2020) 'The global response to the coronavirus: impact on religious practice and religious freedom', Factsheet: Coronavirus, United States Commission on International Religious Freedom, March. Available at www.uscirf.gov/sites/default/files/2020%20Factsheet%20Covid-19%20and%20FoRB.pdf.

Weintraub, R., A. Bitton and M. L. Rosenberg (2020) 'The danger of vaccine nationalism', *Harvard Business Review*, 22 May. Available at https://hbr.org/2020/05/the-danger-of-vaccine-nationalism.

WHO (2020a) 'Advice on the use of masks in the context of COVID-19', Interim Guidance, 6 April. Available at https://apps.who.int/iris/bitstream/handle/10665/331693/WHO-2019-nCov-IPC_Masks-2020.3-eng.pdf?sequence=1&isAllowed=y.

WHO (2020b) 'Advice on the use of masks in the context of COVID-19', Interim Guidance,

5 June. Available at https://apps.who.int/iris/
bitstream/handle/10665/332293/WHO-2019-
nCov-IPC_Masks-2020.4-eng.pdf?
sequence=1&isAllowed=y.

WHO (2020c) 'Mask use in the context of
COVID-19', 1 December. Available at https://
apps.who.int/iris/rest/bitstreams/1319378/
retrieve.

Wieringa, S., D. Dreesens, F. Forland et al.
(2018a) 'Different knowledge, different styles
of reasoning: a challenge for guideline
development', *BMJ Evididence Based
Medicine* 23(3): 87–91. DOI: https://doi.org/
10.1136/bmjebm-2017-110844.

Wieringa, S., E. Engebretsen, K. Heggen and
T. Greenhalgh (2018b) 'Rethinking bias and
truth in evidence-based health care', *Journal
of Evaluation in Clinical Practice* 24(5):
940–938.

Wilkinson, A. (2020) 'The impact of Covid-19 in
informal settlements – are we paying enough
attention?', *Institute of Development Studies*,
17 March. Available at www.ids.ac.uk/opin
ions/the-impact-of-covid-19-in-informal-
settlements-are-we-paying-enough-atten
tion/.

Willingham, E. (2020) 'The condoms of the face:
why some men refuse to wear masks',
Scientific American, 29 June. Available at
www.scientificamerican.com/article/the-
condoms-of-the-face-why-some-men-
refuse-to-wear-masks/.

Wittner, R. (2021) 'Anti-maskers protest outside
Beverly Hills Sephora', *Patch*, 7 April.

Available at https://patch.com/california/bev
erlyhills/anti-maskers-protest-outside-
beverly-hills-sephora.

Wolfe, R. M. and L. K. Sharp (2002) 'Anti-
vaccinationists past and present', *BMJ* 325:
430–432.

Wright, A. (2020) 'Harris study: political
messaging outweighs other factors in face
mask usage', *UChicago News*, 21 October.
Available at https://news.uchicago.edu/story/
who-does-or-doesnt-wear-mask-
partisanship-explains-response-covid-19.

Wright, N. (2020) 'Coronavirus and the future
of surveillance', *Foreign Affairs*, 6 April.
Available at www.foreignaffairs.com/articles/
2020-04-06/coronavirus-and-future-
surveillance.

Young, T. (2021) 'The case against lockdown:
a reply to Christopher Snowdon'. *Quillette*,
5 February. Available at https://quillette.com
/2021/02/05/the-case-against-lockdown-a-re
ply-to-christopher-snowdon/.

Zhang, R, L. Yixin A. L. Zhang, Y. Wang and
M, J. Molina (2020) 'Identifying airborne
transmission as the dominant route for the
spread of COVID-19', *Proceedings of the
National Academy of Sciences of the United
States of America*, 11 June. DOI: https://
doi.org/10.1073/pnas.2009637117.

Zine, J. (2020) 'Unmasking the racial politics of
the coronovirus pandemic', *The Conversation*,
3 June. Available at https://theconversation
.com/unmasking-the-racial-politics-of-the-
coronavirus-pandemic-139011.

Index